The Nice Girl's Guide to
Naughty Sex

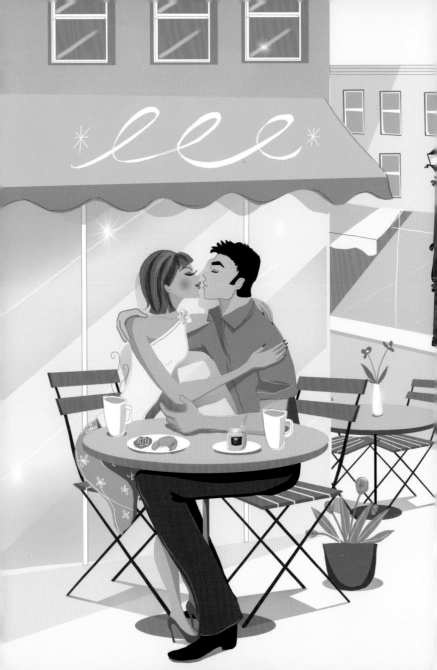

The Nice Girl's Guide to
Naughty Sex

LISA SUSSMAN

Illustrated by
LUCY TRUMAN

Amorata Press

Published by:
AMORATA PRESS,
an imprint of Ulysses Press
P.O. Box 3440
Berkeley, CA 94703
www.amoratapress.com

First published in the U.K. in 2005 as *Sex in the City Day & Night* by Carlton Books Limited

ISBN10: 1-56975-631-7
ISBN13: 978-1-56975-631-7
Library of Congress Control Number: 2007906123

Printed in the United States by Bang Printing

10 9 8 7 6 5 4 3 2 1

Acquisitions Editor: Nick Denton-Brown
Managing Editor: Claire Chun
Editorial and production staff: Lauren Harrison, Amy Hough, Lisa Kester, Judith Metzener, Elyce Petker, Abby Reser, Emma Silvers
Cover design: DiAnna VanEyke
Interior design & layout: what!design @ whatweb.com

Distributed by Publishers Group West

This book has been written and published strictly for informational purposes, and in no way should it be used as a substitute for consultation with professional therapists. All facts in this book came from scientific publications, personal interviews, published trade books, self-published materials by experts, magazine articles, and the personal-practice experiences of the authorities quoted or sources cited. The author and publisher are providing you with information in this work so that you can have the knowledge and can choose, at your own risk, to act on that knowledge.

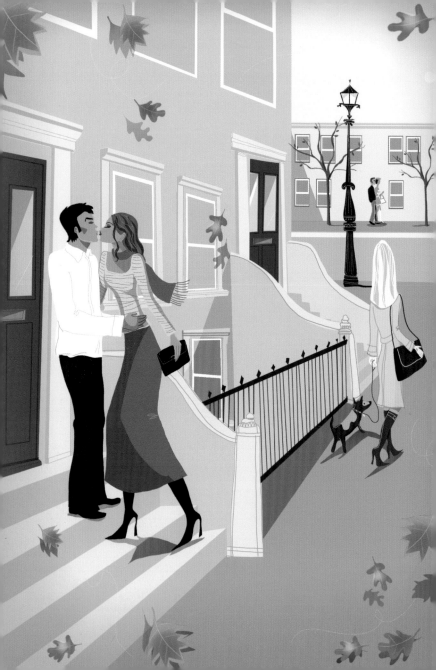

Introduction

Let's get one thing straight: there is nothing wrong with being a nice girl. You're every man's dream, right? So go right on being the girl he's proud to take to his company's picnic and his parents' house for the holidays.

On the other hand, just because you melt his heart by baking him a cake on his birthday doesn't mean you can't also light a fire lower down later that night. So if you're a little too nice in the one place where it pays to be naughty, this book comes to your rescue. Get ready for more passionate positions, sensual scenarios and inspiring ideas than you ever thought possible.

A little nookie know-how is not a dangerous thing, especially if it adds a little more "omg" to your orgasms. So at the end of the day (or earlier if you two just can't wait), give the nice girl a night off and let your inner sex goddess out to play. With the between-the-sheets sexperiments in this book, you can make his and your own naughty dreams come true.

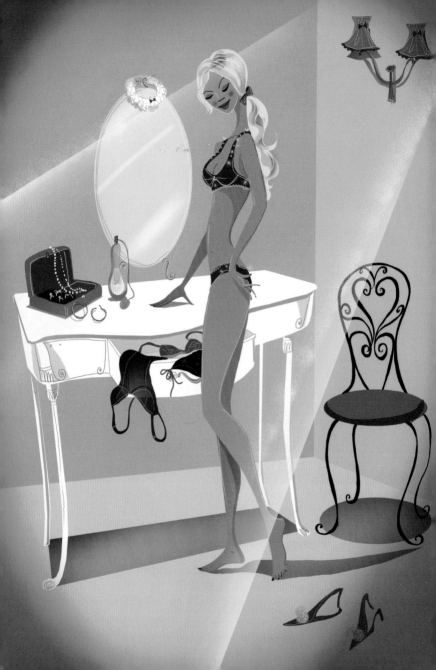

Foreplay

You know how he always skips the instructions. If something says "Read Before Opening," he just tears into it right away. That approach might even work during sex—for the guys. To make sex great for both of you, you need to slow things down. In addition to the ideas in this chapter, consider these tantalizing techniques that you both can enjoy:

1. **Touch each other through your clothing** rather than heading straight for skin-to-skin action. You might even be able to get away with this in public.

2. **Explore uncharted erogenous zones**—upper thighs, behind the knees, the neck and the area just below the belly button.

3. **Learn to be ambidextrous.** While you massage your lover's hot spots with one hand, work on your own pleasure center with your other hand.

4. **Make noise.** Talk dirty if you want, but even simple moans let him know when he is doing something right.

Sweet Sex

Forget chocolate instead of sex—chocolate is best when mixed with sex. Chocolate contains both serotonin and phenylethylamine, chemicals that make your brain feel like the love bug has bitten it. Eat enough chocolate, and your heart races, your blood pressure rises and you feel a happy buzz. Luckily for your diet, you only need a little bit of the stuff to add a bit more zing to your love life.

* Leave a trail of heart-shaped chocolates from the front door to the bed with a note about the events planned.

* Hand-feed each other freshly dipped chocolate-covered strawberries. Don't worry about drips—you can lick them off afterward!

* Drip warm melted chocolate all over each other's bodies and slowly lap it up.

* Smear each other with chocolate fudge, chocolate ice cream and chocolate sprinkles to make a human sundae—yum.

* Share a bar of chocolate after lovemaking. Who knows—if chocolate's aphrodisiac qualities are to be believed, you may be ready for another go sooner than you anticipated!

Bite Me

There's nothing more erotic than a partner who knows where and how to give love bites. He can nibble at your shoulders and neck when he drapes his body over yours and slips in from behind. You can reciprocate as you cozy up during afterplay.

WATCH OUT!!! Don't bite so hard that you leave identifying tooth marks.

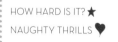

HOW HARD IS IT? ★

NAUGHTY THRILLS ♥

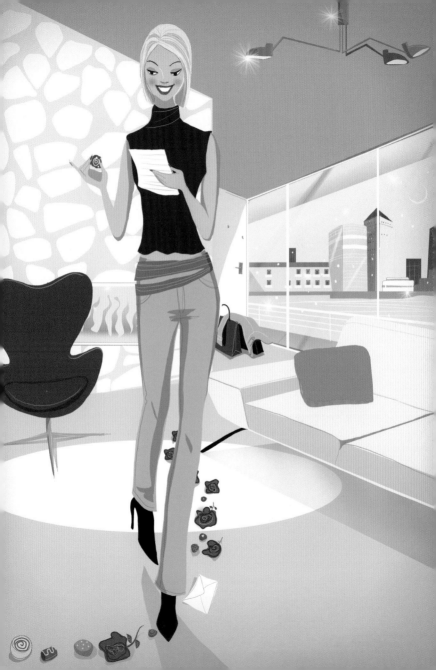

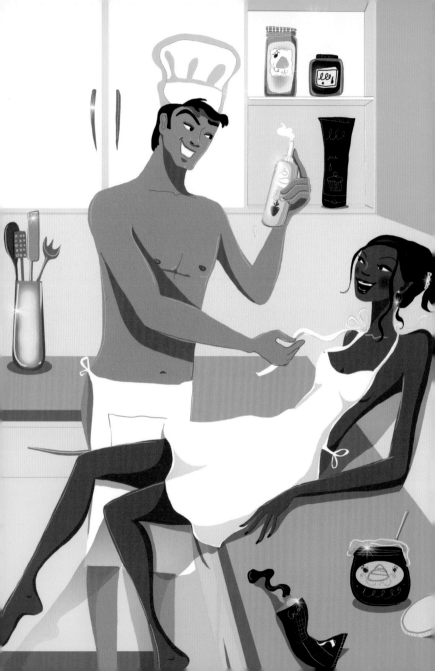

Tasty Turn-Ons

Indulge in a tasty turn-on. Lay cuddling in a side-by-side position and slip berries or pieces of mango back and forth between your mouths.

HOW HARD IS IT? ★
NAUGHTY THRILLS ♥

Whipped Cream Bikini

The whipped cream bikini is the adult male equivalent of the Happy Meal: It's the food that comes with a toy.

NICE & EASY: You can take the can and decorate yourself or let your partner be the pastry chef.

HOW HARD IS IT? ★
NAUGHTY THRILLS ♥

EXTRA NAUGHTY: A squirt of chocolate sauce on top makes it even tastier.

Going Down on Him

You know that men love it when you give them a blowjob. But it can be uncomfortable, neck-aching, throat-choking work (why do they call it a job, after all?). Luckily, all it takes is a simple adjustment of position to make you—and him—bob for joy. If you kneel in front of him while he sits on the sofa, you'll be able to control the depth of penetration and keep your gag reflex in check. All you need to do is take his lollipop into your mouth and suck to give a basic blowjob that he will love. If you want to upgrade your oral fixation, use lots of spit to make it wet and slippery, move up and down instead of just sucking, and probe the head with a stiff tongue.

HOW HARD IS IT? ★★

NAUGHTY THRILLS ♥♥ *(for him)*

WATCH OUT!!! To prevent gagging while pleasuring him, you can hold the base of his joystick while you suck. This controls how deeply he goes into your mouth.

There is such a thing as the perfect blowjob—the key is to realize that he does not want to be licked the way you do. He is into a quicker rhythm with lots of sucking movements. To get started, lie on your back with your head on a pillow, while he dangles himself above you, supporting his weight on his arms. This way he will control the action. The trick is not to gobble him like a seal swallowing a herring, but to use a hard sucking motion.

WATCH OUT!!! The only mistake you can make is to use too little or too much pressure—the same energy used to suck on a lollipop is about right.

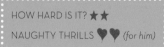

HOW HARD IS IT? ★★

NAUGHTY THRILLS ♥♥ *(for him)*

He stands and you kneel at his love altar. This is such a hot fantasy for most guys that you don't even have to pay homage for long.

NICE & EASY: What's actually best about this move is that it lets you use your whole body to move your mouth back and forth on him, so your neck doesn't get tired. Plus you can pull yourself back if he gets pushy and tries to move in too deep.

HOW HARD IS IT? ★
NAUGHTY THRILLS 💜 💜 *(for him)*

EXTRA NAUGHTY: This move also leaves your hands free so you can use them on the boys.

Blame the movies, but no man feels his life is complete unless he has been deep-throated at least once. The problem is that the average throat is not made for swallowing a 6-8 inch sausage whole (yes, guys—that really is the standard measurement). To turn your throat into a love passage, you will need to lie back on the bed and hang your head off the edge. He can then stand by the side so that his penis is lined up with your mouth.

NICE & EASY: You can use your hands against his thighs to control action.

EXTRA NAUGHTY: This is actually a good position for you to practice your

HOW HARD IS IT? ★ ★ ★
NAUGHTY THRILLS 💜 💜 💜
and then some (for him)

gargling skills and swallowing when he shoots. The reason most women gag is because their throat muscles are tight with the expectation of what's to—er—come. But in this position, the throat muscles are too stretched to tense up.

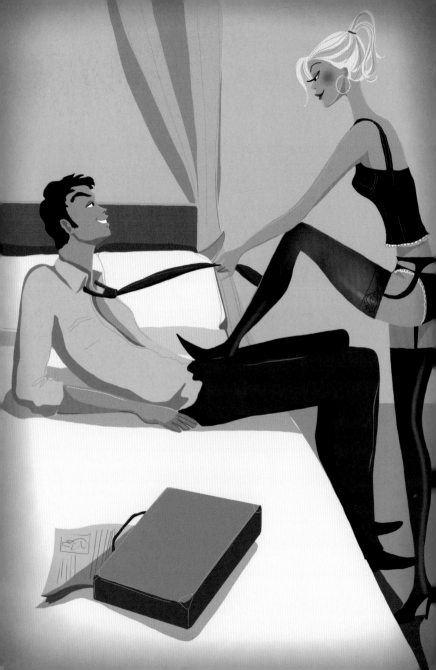

Mistress at Home

HOW HARD IS IT? ★
NAUGHTY THRILLS ♥ ♥ ♥

You saunter out in spiked heels, a black garter belt and a pair of silk thigh-high stockings. Make sure he gets the full power of your passion by aggressively pushing him back on the bed before he gets a chance to undress. Loosen his belt and climb on top.

NICE & EASY: If he is wearing a tie, hold onto it like he's a dog on a leash to remind him who's in charge.

EXTRA NAUGHTY: You should keep your gear on the whole time.

Barely There

HOW HARD IS IT? ★ ★ ★
NAUGHTY THRILLS ♥ ♥

You meet and greet him wearing only a long coat over your birthday suit. If in public, you should drag him off to a private corner, but if you flash him at home, do it right there against the front door. You stand with your legs spread. He inserts one slightly bent leg between yours. This will give you something to balance against in case he needs to raise you up a bit to match up your love anatomy.

EXTRA NAUGHTY: You can also grind your hips so that his upper thigh pushes against your clitoris.

Going Down on Her

Many women find oral sex a more guaranteed method of climaxing than actual intercourse. He can make the most of it by winding his tongue up and giving you an all-over body bath. The

HOW HARD IS IT? ★ ★ ★

NAUGHTY THRILLS ♥ ♥ ♥ *(cubed for you)*

best position for this is on your back with your legs bent. He works from above, giving TLC (Tongue Licking Care) to your erogenous zones: belly, inner thighs, behind the knees, feet, bottom and the area surrounding your genitals. He can make you really squirm by working his lips around your love box but holding back before giving you a tongue lashing.

EXTRA NAUGHTY: Place a pillow under your buttocks to change the angle. He can then reacquaint himself with parts already visited.

Straight lapping gives cunnilingus a bad name. If he doesn't want to get "The Tap" (a rap on the shoulder to say, "Enough, I might as well be getting waxed for all the pleasure you're giving me"), he should avoid sucking you up like a Hoover or any tongue-lapping that makes

HOW HARD IS IT? ★ ★

NAUGHTY THRILLS ♥ ♥ ♥ *(for you)*

your vagina feel like it's getting a pummelling. Help him develop a variety of different moves. Have him tease the clitoris with quick, short licks, give your love button a French kiss, then nibble gently. Ask him to swoop his tongue in long, lazy figure eights, meandering around your edges, crisscrossing your lips and pausing each time to press on your horn.

EXTRA NAUGHTY: He can multitask by using both his fingers and his tongue, sticking one up the vaginal canal while the other works your love knob or pokes around your asshole.

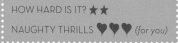
Most men will perform oral sex in one of two positions: with you lying on your back or in classic number 69. To break the rut, sit on the edge of a chair (better than a sofa, which you may end up staining if you're a gusher). You can use the chair's support to lean back, your bottom on the edge and your legs wide open so he can come on in.

EXTRA NAUGHTY: He can use his tongue to trace letters on your na-na—it'll add to the moment for you and keep his interest going (can he spell "touchdown"?).

You don't always have to lie back and take it. For some wild animal, mouth-to-vagina loving, both partners get on all fours, you in front so your na-na is in front of his face. This will give him a different angle to work from than the one he usually gets with you on your back. Old dogs at the oral game know it's not enough just to whip out his tongue and lap at your bone until you are ready to play dead. He'll need to sniff around and work in a few different motions to get your tail wagging. First, he should use only the tip of his tongue and do a quick up and down motion hitting right on the clitoris. Next, have him twiddle his tongue around your clitoris in circles. He can work clockwise and then reverse directions. Finally, you will want him to do a rowdy, anything-goes motion where he twists his tongue, turns it and swishes it back and forth.

NICE & EASY: You'll eventually need a simple rhythm focusing on your love knot to take you all the way to a capital "O."

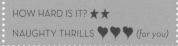

Rubdown

Soothe those sore muscles with an erotic massage. All you need is a coin to toss to decide who goes first. The person receiving (called Lucky Bastard from now on) lies flat on their back. The person massaging (hereafter known as Slave) straddles the Lucky Bastard's tummy and rubs with long, gliding strokes.

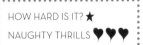

HOW HARD IS IT? ★

NAUGHTY THRILLS ♥ ♥ ♥

The human body is full of parts that need to be kneaded, so don't skip ahead to your favorite spots just yet. Make sure to work these areas first:

SIDES Work your way up and down from just underneath the armpits to the hips, using long, slow, continuous strokes with the palms of your open hands. If they feel ticklish, it means you're going too fast and not deep enough.

SACRUM This is the bony plate where the spine meets the bottom, and it's absolutely packed with sensitive nerve endings. Use your fingers to rub its surface and don't be afraid to dig your fingers in.

PULSE POINTS Find them under the earlobes and just under the jawbone (feel for the pulse, which hopefully is already racing). Rubbing in light, tiny circles with three fingers will send a message to the brain that it's show time.

TOES Applying pressure with your thumb, trace a line from the top of the big toe down into the webbing between it and the second toe. Continue up the second toe and so on, repeating the movement all the way down to the little toe.

Now you are ready for the main attraction. The Slave moves their chest over the Lucky Bastard's, lightly brushing them with their nipples, moving side to side and up and down. The Slave then opens the Lucky Bastard's legs and slides between them to gently massage their love muscles until they melt.

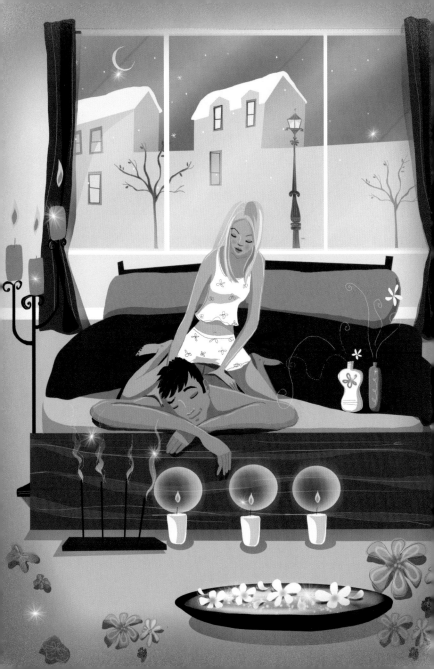

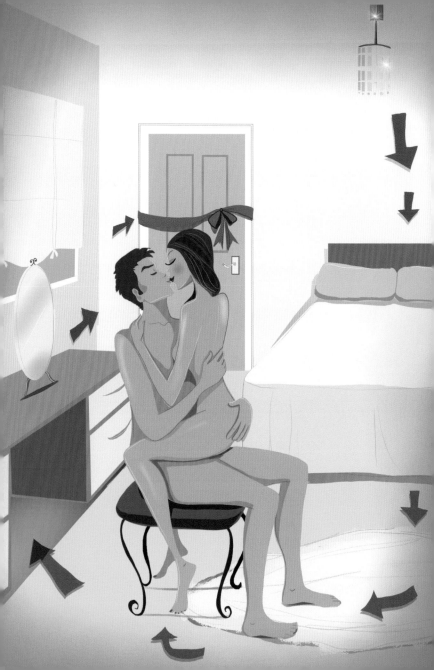

In the Bedroom

Your bedroom doesn't have to be a bored room. Think of your love nest as more than a bed–it's the perfect place for improving your nookie know-how during long, passionate lovemaking. To get it in shape for these sexathons, you should first give your bedroom a naughty makeover that will create more of a passion buzz.

1. Relocate your least sexy stuff outside of the bedroom. An elegant dressing table is fine, but keep your beauty products in the bathroom, clothes in the closet and stuffed animal collection hidden from view.

2. Make your bed the center of attention. Don't smash it in a corner or against a back wall. Leave at least three sides free for over-the-edge frolicking.

3. Add a few mirrors to your decor. Just don't be crass and hang one above the bed. Mirrors improve any room and, if carefully placed, can add some visual sizzle to your spicy scenarios.

4. Dim the lights. Create a more romantic atmosphere by installing bulbs with as low a wattage as possible. And don't be afraid to use colored bulbs as well. A bedroom with hues of pink will be true to your nice girl heart. As your room warms up, so will his passion.

All Day in Bed

 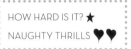
Prolong your passion and intensify your sex session by spending all day in bed.

* Skip washing the dishes, answering the phone or even getting dressed.

* Stock up on a feast of treats for a bed picnic—fruit, cheese, bread, chocolate, fresh juice and a bottle of bubbly.

* Set the mood with scented candles, comfy cushions and sexy tunes.

* Turn the bed into a love cocoon with silk bedding.

Do It on the Floor

 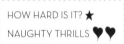
Doing it on the floor next to the bed makes you feel so sexy and urgent about your pleasure that you can't even wait to roll onto the mattress. Unless the floor is covered with a rug you'll want to do your mambo standing up—you lean on your elbows against the bed while he comes up from behind. Once he's in, you can lift one leg to suck him in even deeper.

NICE & EASY: He can help by holding the lifted leg.

Once you get going, go slow. Having slo-mo sex will make the exquisite agony last for at least a few hours. Lie on your sides with him curled up behind you. He slides his penis inside you, as slowly as possible, while you both focus on the feeling of your skin making contact and on the pleasurable pressure of his slowly advancing penis. Take a full minute to perform what you would usually do in just one or two seconds. Slo-mo sex will make you acutely aware of every move, from the muscles and body parts you're using to your weight shifts and your breathing—all of which you fail to notice when you move quickly.

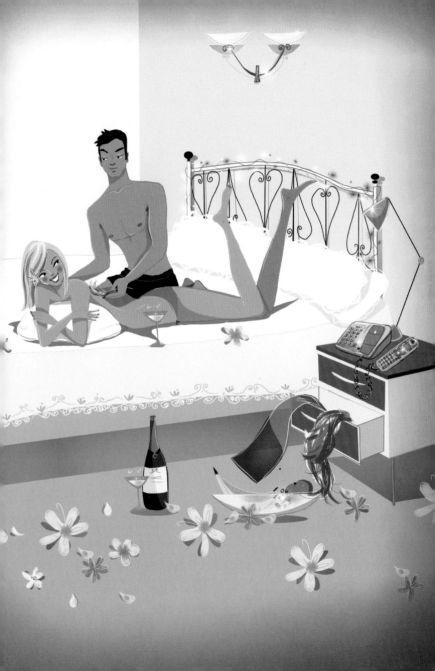

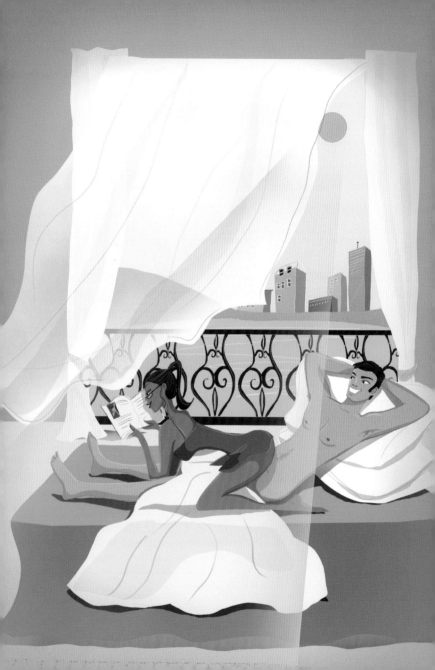

More Bedroom Time

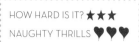

HOW HARD IS IT? ★ ★ ★

NAUGHTY THRILLS ♥ ♥ ♥

Let's face it, when it comes to making sex last, he's the problem. The average man is ready to call it a night after one orgasm. To increase his staying power, slip into missionary, since this is the position that gives him the most control. When he feels that he's about to reach the point of no return, he contracts his PC muscle hard for five seconds. The result: all the great feelings of orgasm without the ejaculation, and he will still have his stiffy.

Triple X Story Hour

Take turns getting on top and reading erotic stories to each other—whoever is in the upper position sits and reads.

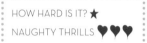

HOW HARD IS IT? ★

NAUGHTY THRILLS ♥ ♥ ♥

WATCH OUT!!! Be prepared to toss the book to the side and let your urges take over.

Swinging in the Bedroom

This move is as close as you can get to having sex in a swing set without having to install the actual hardware in your bedroom. He leans his

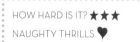

HOW HARD IS IT? ★ ★ ★

NAUGHTY THRILLS ♥

shoulders back against the bed or a wall with his feet on the floor, supporting the bulk of his weight, in a chair position. You straddle his midsection and use your legs to thrust.

Missionary

Get into basic missionary, but don't stop there. Raise your legs so that your knees are pressed to your chest and your calves are draped over his shoulders. This will make your vagina longer, which will make his toes curl as he can penetrate you more deeply and give you more friction and pressure where you crave it the most—your vaginal lips and clitoris.

HOW HARD IS IT? ★★

NAUGHTY THRILLS ♥♥♥

EXTRA NAUGHTY: Instead of just grinding into you, he should slide forward and up. This will boost the friction on her outtie.

Your true love gets on top of you in missionary and holds his upper body away from you at an angle. You then spread your legs wide open, bend your knees and grab hold of your ankles, making sure that your arms are inside your legs. Use your elbows to push the sides of your knees as far down

HOW HARD IS IT? ★★★

NAUGHTY THRILLS ♥♥

to the mattress as you can get them. Your knees should be pointed out, not up. As he begins to take the plunge, you hold your ankles firm and press down harder on your knees—the flatter you can get your legs, the more intense the sensation. You then thrust yourself up to meet him as he grinds down. This move allows you to be as wide open as possible and feel every inch of him penetrating you.

NICE & EASY: You can put your feet on the sides of his bottom to better station your ankles.

Once he's inside you, bring your legs close together and have him hook his ankles around your calves, then raise himself up slightly on his hands with a small arch in his back. By closing your legs, you will create a more snug entry for him and more continuous clitoral stimulation for you—his groin will be doing a rumba on your hot spot.

NICE & EASY: Tighten your lower muscles (your hips, glutes and thighs) to create rhythmic clenching in your pelvic area for an orgasmic blast-off.

For those who have done it, seen it and bought the T-shirt, there's the Body Twist. You lie back with your legs up, open and wide apart while he lowers

himself onto you, face down and lying with his legs on either side of your shoulders. Rest your legs on his back while he thrusts backward.

You lie on your back and lift your legs so they're over your ears and parallel to the floor. He kneels in front of you, butting his knees against your lower back to support you. He then leans his body up against your thighs, dips in and gently rocks them both back and forth.

NICE & EASY: He bends forward to slip you a love peck, which drives his jackhammer even deeper.

EXTRA NAUGHTY: For a tight fit, raise your legs from behind your head to straight up in the air, as high as possible.

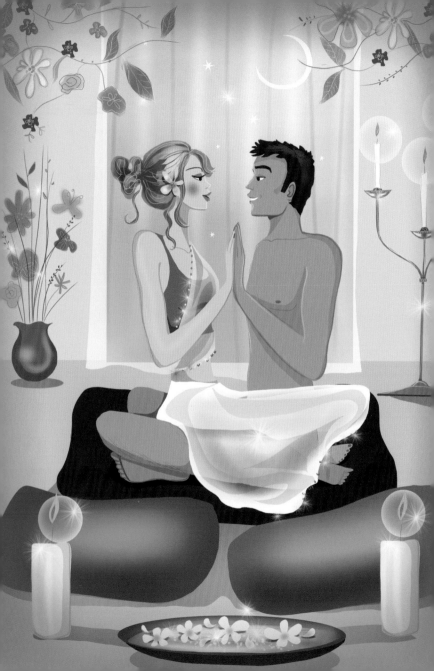

Say Ooohmm!

Western sex is focused on having an orgasm, while Eastern sex looks at sex as something larger to share—a deeper, more divine sexperience. Love made Eastern-style can last hours (read: hours of pure soul-in-sync bliss—mmmm).

Agree with your partner that you won't try to start having intercourse until you've toyed with each other for a full 60 minutes.

First, face each other standing and slowly strip each other's clothes off. Take at least five minutes with each piece of clothing, pausing to stroke any body part that is revealed.

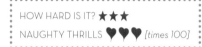

HOW HARD IS IT? ★ ★ ★

NAUGHTY THRILLS ♥ ♥ ♥ [times 100]

Now begins what the Taoists call "the time of the K'ang," which is Chinese for "bed." Slide between the sheets, kissing each other and taking deep, relaxing breaths in tandem.

For the next 25 minutes, neither of you should do anything but kiss and caress the non-hot zones of each other's bodies. Spend five minutes kissing just each other's nipples. Practice eye-rousal. Gaze into each other's peepers for at least a minute.

In the remaining 25 minutes of the hour, move on to stroking the sexual areas. But the Tao belief is: Don't rush!

Then, sit facing one another and wrap your legs around each other's backs. Snuggle in by grasping each other's elbows and leaning in to hold each other's weight—this will keep you in place. Now, holding hands, see if you can tilt your heads far enough back to rest them on the floor. Try to remain still and concentrate on your bodies connecting and the sexual energies flowing through you both.

The Meditation

Tantrics embrace each other's aura (the energy fields said to buzz around each person) for full-body orgasms. Start by imagining yourselves encircled in a glowing orb of light. Now, facing each other in a seated or standing position, he puts his Arrow of Love (figure it out) in her Seat of Pleasure. Don't move—instead, concentrate on breathing and looking into each other's eyes. Try to hold out for 30 minutes—the result will be cosmic.

WATCH OUT!!! If he seems like he is about to wilt from the heat, you can jiggle your hips and give him a squeeze to pump him back to life.

The Three-Pointed Star

You lie on your back on the floor with your left leg extended straight up in the air and your right leg stretched out to your right, perpendicular to your body. Reaching out across the floor with your right hand, you clasp your right knee, forming a triangle with your right side, right leg and right arm. He crouches at the bottom and enters your galaxy.

NICE & EASY: This crouching position boosts his pelvic control so he'll be able to touch you in ways you've never felt before.

The Jumping Frog

Start in standard missionary position. He then rises up on all fours, and you raise your pelvis to meet his penis. As he stays stationary, you start moving your hips up and down to get things jumping.

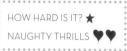

HOW HARD IS IT? ★

NAUGHTY THRILLS 🖤 🖤

NICE & EASY: Although you're on the bottom, you call the shots here—by lifting your pelvis, you can control the speed and timing of every thrust according to your wanton whims. This is the Tantric position for making sure you get your "O" on.

EXTRA NAUGHTY: You can tease him mercilessly by thrusting only halfway onto him. This will centralize all sensations on the super-sensitive tip of his yang.

Set of Nines

Tao teaches that a man can train himself to bring a woman to an orgasmic big bang by entering her with a thousand (that's right—one thousand) strokes. In this

HOW HARD IS IT? ★ ★

NAUGHTY THRILLS 🖤 🖤 🖤

considerably reduced version, he slides into missionary and enters you with nine shallow thrusts (the head of his penis just tickles your vagina), withdraws, pauses and then re-enters, thrusting shallowly and quickly eight times, pushing inside for one last deep thrust. This thrust-and-rest routine continues for seven shallow and two deep, six shallow and three deep, and so on until you both collapse in a quivering heap on the ninth thrusting stroke.

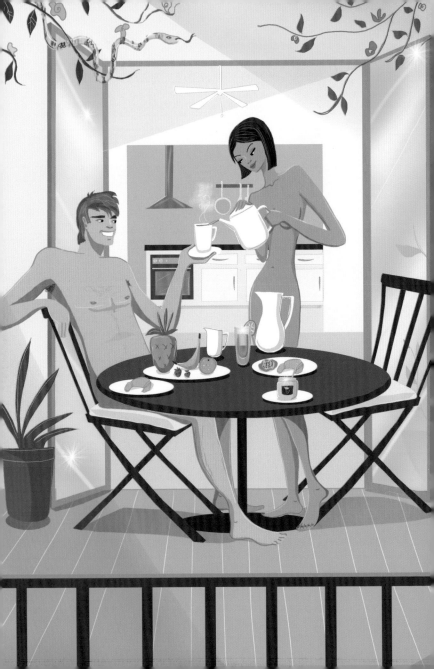

Around the House

Nothing turns up the heat faster than having sex out of the bedroom. So put your furnace on high and watch your whole house get hot.

While any room can be an arena for an athletic romp, **the living room** is the easiest place to migrate. With a sofa and soft rugs serving as a bed-like playing field, you'll discover that you don't need to master any new skills for this game.

The next rooms to explore are the **kitchen** and **dining room**. But a word of warning: Do not expect candlelit, soft-focused, romantic dinner sex. With high counters and solid table tops, you're going to find your feet dangling above the floor while you're floating on cloud nine.

You don't want to wait too long before moving on to the **bathroom**, since sex in the tub combines heat, pressure, moisture and friction—all in one steamy place. Not to mention that doing it in the water makes you feel lighter than a soap bubble. So get ready to lather up.

Don't stop with the just the big rooms, either. Look all over your house, from the **washer** and **dryer** to the **stairs** and **windows**, and you'll find plenty of nooks and crannies for spontaneous hanky panky.

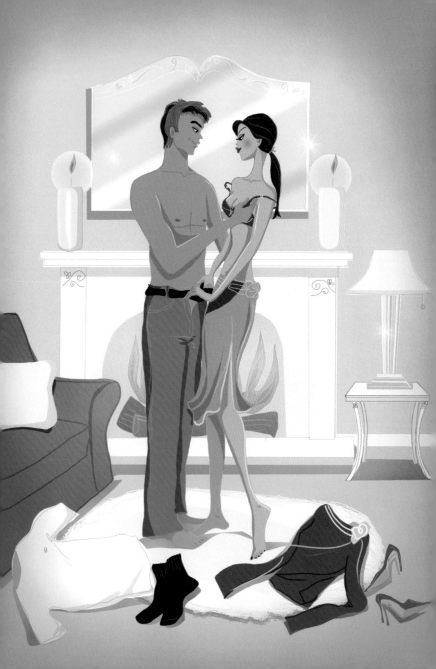

The Sofa

He sits back on the sofa while you straddle his lap with your legs splayed apart and your knees bent up against his chest. You then lean back so you're almost upside-down, your arms stretched behind you (all the way to the floor) to support your weight.

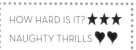

HOW HARD IS IT? ★ ★ ★
NAUGHTY THRILLS ♥ ♥

NICE & EASY: Open and close your legs and give him a few good squeezes.

EXTRA NAUGHTY: When you're ready for him to hit his passion peak, you should give a final power squeeze when he's completely inside to send him soaring.

Fuzzy Feelings

HOW HARD IS IT? ★
NAUGHTY THRILLS ♥ ♥

There's nothing like rolling around on something soft and fuzzy to make you purr with pleasure. Turn your living room into a bear's lair and release your inner wild animal. Spread a faux fur rug in front of a crackling fire, dim the lights, and get cozy. Don't worry about getting too close to the flames: you'll have no choice. Lie canoodling in a spooning position so you both can get the furry feeling.

Dining Table

You sit on the work surface with your legs spread-eagle, he faces you and plunges deep inside.

NICE & EASY: Cover the table with a cloth first to make it more comfortable.

EXTRA NAUGHTY: This is a fairly comfy position so take your time. Reach for some food—pile anything that can be licked off within easy reach (whipped cream, ice cream, sweet sauces). Think of it as dessert.

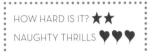

HOW HARD IS IT? ★★

NAUGHTY THRILLS ♥♥♥

WATCH OUT!!! Make sure you give the table a good wash before inviting any guests over for dinner.

Kitchen Counter

You sit on the work surface, he stands in front of you and you wrap your legs around him. The angle means that he goes in deep and nuzzles your G-spot, so you'll create mega heat in minimal time.

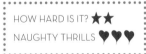

HOW HARD IS IT? ★★

NAUGHTY THRILLS ♥♥♥

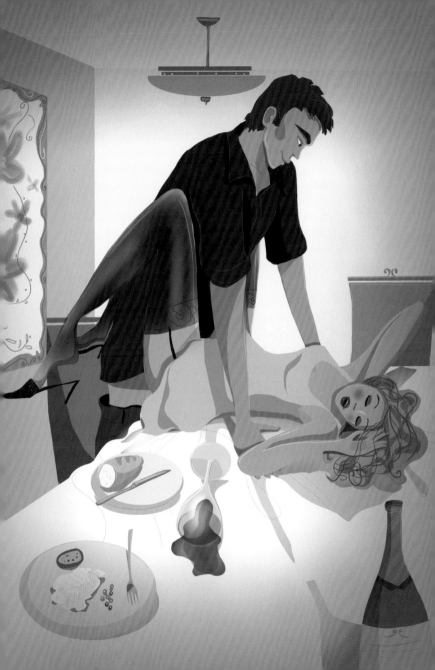

Kitchen Sink

He lifts you up onto the edge of the kitchen sink and enters you from the front (he may have to stand on a low stool to get in the scene). Turn the water on (nice and warm) and let it spray on your back and bottom.

NICE & EASY: If your sink has a nozzle spray, direct the jets of water over each other for a vibe-like buzz.

WATCH OUT!!! Make sure you test the water before you start or you could end up scalding each other—that's not the kind of heat you're looking for.

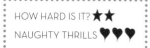
HOW HARD IS IT? ★★
NAUGHTY THRILLS ♥♥♥

Kitchen Chair

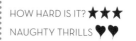
HOW HARD IS IT? ★★★
NAUGHTY THRILLS ♥♥

Those straight-backed chairs actually give a lot of maneuvering room so you can have a full love menu. You can sit on his lap facing away from him and then twist around mid-action to face him, wrapping your legs around him. Or you can simply kneel or stand facing the chair and he can come in from behind.

WATCH OUT!!! For the last move you will need to hold onto the back of the chair or you may topple over when things (hopefully) get vigorous.

Office Chair

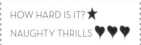

HOW HARD IS IT? ★

NAUGHTY THRILLS ♥ ♥ ♥

Swivel chairs are perfect for going south. You sit down and he takes his place on the floor in front of you. He then gets to work with his tongue while he moves you–chair and all–side to side. After you recover, you can return the favor.

EXTRA NAUGHTY: Don't deadline your orgasm. Take your time. Beat around the bush. Tease and mix it up with nibbles and licks as well as laps. You want the other person at the edge of the seat, not asleep in it.

WATCH OUT!!! If the seat is leather or covered with a light fabric, you may want to cover it with a towel before starting your tongue-lashing.

Office Desk

You lie back so your bottom is at the edge, while he stands in front of you. You then lift your legs and rest your feet on his shoulders. Now the hard part: you tilt your pelvis upwards so that your back forms a straight line angling up toward him and your crotches meet and greet. Now watch the friction build.

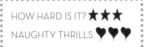

HOW HARD IS IT? ★ ★ ★

NAUGHTY THRILLS ♥ ♥ ♥

NICE & EASY: He should put his hands just under your hips so that he can hold your booty at the perfect angle while he thrusts into you.

WATCH OUT!!! This move is deep and rubs in all the right places, so expect a body shaking orgasm, which means you probably want to make sure the computer, phone and any important papers have been shoved to the other side of the desk before you start.

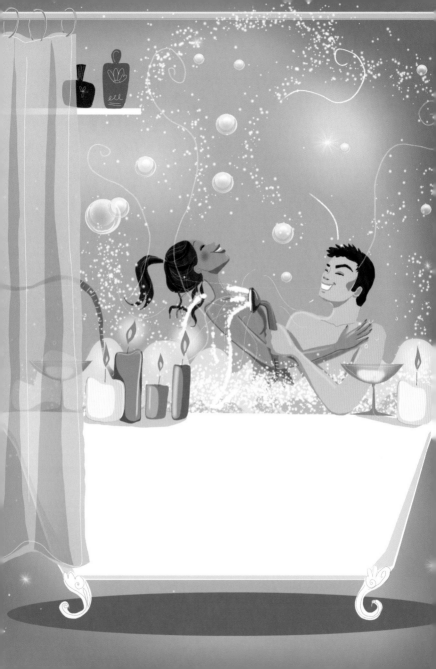

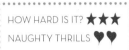
Bath

HOW HARD IS IT? ★ ★ ★
NAUGHTY THRILLS ♥ ♥

Making love in the bath can be a deliciously dirty sexperience, but bathrooms were not well designed for sex. The lighting in bathrooms isn't generally sympathetic to romance, so save on electricity and use scented candles. Place them around the edge of the bath and light them while the bath is still filling so their sensuous scent perfumes the air.

It can also be a tight squeeze if you don't have a large tub. Fortunately, this move is one-size-fits-all. Fill the bath halfway with hot water. He gets in first with his back to one end of the bath, holding himself up by propping his hands behind him, on the edge of the tub. His legs should be spread out in front of him with his knees slightly bent.

Now you get in, sitting so that your arms are propping you up behind you in the same position as his and your legs are bent on either side of his hips (if the bath isn't big enough to get a stable surface, just wrap them around his waist). Slip him in, using your hand. Don't worry if he slips out—the buoyancy of the water means that it'll probably take a few tries before you can get going, but that's part of what makes it such an intensely hot experience! Once he's securely in place, keep your movements small and slow. Go with the flow, using the motion of the water to rock you up and down.

NICE & EASY: You can push your bottom forward and lift your hips a few inches to help him find your plug.

WATCH OUT!!! A woman's natural lubrication will often be washed away when making love in a wet place, so use a silicone-based lubrication—they're waterproof and will last for hours. The only question is, can you?

Side by Side

Lie on your side with him lying down facing you. He then straddles your bottom leg and you rest your top leg around his waist. You should fit together like apple pie and ice cream.

NICE & EASY: To maximize your momentum, he should grab your thigh like it's a javelin he's about to throw and pull you against him when he thrusts.

HOW HARD IS IT? ★★

NAUGHTY THRILLS ♥

EXTRA NAUGHTY LEVEL ONE: He can slowly rotate his hips in a circle, like he's stirring your pudding.

EXTRA NAUGHTY AGAIN: He can pull you open by raising your leg higher and giving you everything he's got.

Fork your bodies into a spooning position. But instead of slipping into a cozy cuddle, reach your hands through your legs to sneak attack on the part of his stiffy not able to get inside of you. He can easily reach all your favorite spots with a little arm stretch.

WATCH OUT!!! When you up the pleasure quotient with add-ons, it can be hard maintaining this position (especially when he starts jumping all over the bed with

HOW HARD IS IT? ★★

NAUGHTY THRILLS ♥ ♥

delight at the double thrill of getting a hand job while having sex). You can keep his erection from pole-vaulting and make him declare undying love at the same time with a tight squeeze.

With this spooning move, he will flip your ON switch with multiple motions. You lie on your side (bottom facing him), then he kneels behind your slightly spread legs so

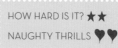

he can enter your love nest from behind. As he thrusts, he uses his left hand to play "X marks the spot" with your love button while stroking your back gently with his right hand. He won't have to keep the triple action going for long before you start begging him not to stop.

NICE & EASY: His left knee should be touching behind your thighs, his right knee right behind your back.

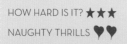

Lie on your side with one bent arm propping up your head. Keep your bottom leg stretched straight down and extend the other straight up in the air so that your two legs form an "L." He then straddles you, facing in the direction of your head (rather than your feet). He can stay seated or edge his way down so that he is also lying on his side facing you.

NICE & EASY: You can rest your top leg on his shoulder.

EXTRA NAUGHTY: You can raise and lower your upper leg to help push him in and out. This will have the added bonus of hitting every sizzle spot between your legs.

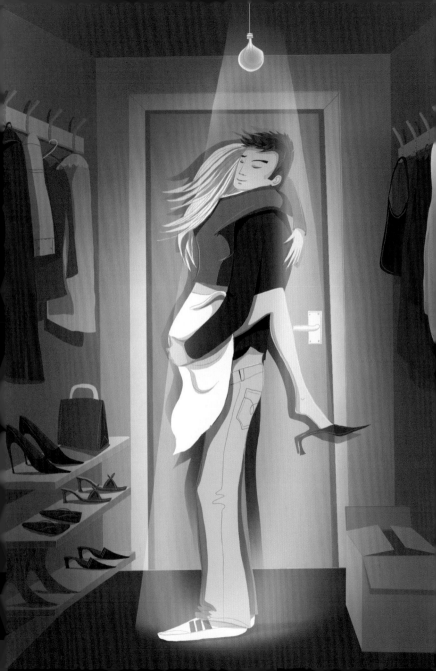

Shower

You brace yourself with your hands on the shower walls and he enters from behind. Be careful not to slip on the soap—this is one you definitely don't want to explain in the hospital.

HOW HARD IS IT? ★
NAUGHTY THRILLS ♥ ♥

NICE & EASY: He may have to bend his knees to get a good plunge angle.

The Closet

The next time you're having a big party, slip away for some private time in your coat closet. Don't get undressed—just pull up your skirt and have standing sex. Re-adjust and return to your guests.

HOW HARD IS IT? ★
NAUGHTY THRILLS ♥ ♥

Washer/Dryer 1

You have a super-sized built-in sex toy in your house: your washer and tumble dryer. He sits on the lid and you sit on top of him (he can keep

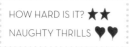

HOW HARD IS IT? ★★

NAUGHTY THRILLS ♥♥

you in place by encircling you in his arms). Flip on the spin cycle. The motion will be transmitted through his pelvis, essentially turning his member into a life-size vibrator.

NICE & EASY: Run a warm-water load so the top won't be cold.

EXTRA NAUGHTY: Select the cottons cycle for the best results. It's a warm wash so his booty won't get cold, plus it has the longest, fastest spin.

Washer/Dryer 2

A variation on the above is for you to sit on top of the machine while he gets between your legs. Washing machines weren't built with this purpose in mind, so you may need a step stool. Commence the wash cycle.

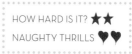

HOW HARD IS IT? ★★

NAUGHTY THRILLS ♥♥

NICE & EASY 1: He should hold your shoulders firmly but lovingly to keep you upright. This maximizes contact between you and the machine's surface. When things heat up, he should press down on your hips so you receive the full effect of the washer's vibrations.

NICE & EASY 2: FYI, you can also do this one on your own.

Door Jam

Pretend there's an earthquake and position yourself in the doorframe. The more narrow the area, the better for positioning yourselves. He leans backward against one side of the door jam and you do the same with the opposite side, straddling him first. Hold onto the frame behind you with your hands and press your bottom against the surface to stay in place as you gently thrust your way in and out of your house.

EXTRA NAUGHTY: Use your front door, where the possibility of getting caught by neighbors or housemates adds to the thrill.

WATCH OUT!!! Wear shoes or go barefoot—socks can make things slippery.

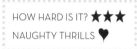

HOW HARD IS IT? ★ ★ ★

NAUGHTY THRILLS ♥

Stairs

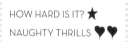

HOW HARD IS IT? ★

NAUGHTY THRILLS ♥ ♥

You can do it coming or going. The stairs are the ideal place for doing it standing and facing each other, since you can stand one step higher than him to line up your love parts.

When you get to the bottom stair, turn your action around. You kneel in front of him at the landing of the staircase, both of you facing the stairs. He holds your hips and walks up your passageway from behind.

WATCH OUT!!! He should hold onto the hand rail or your thrusting may send him toppling backward down the stairs.

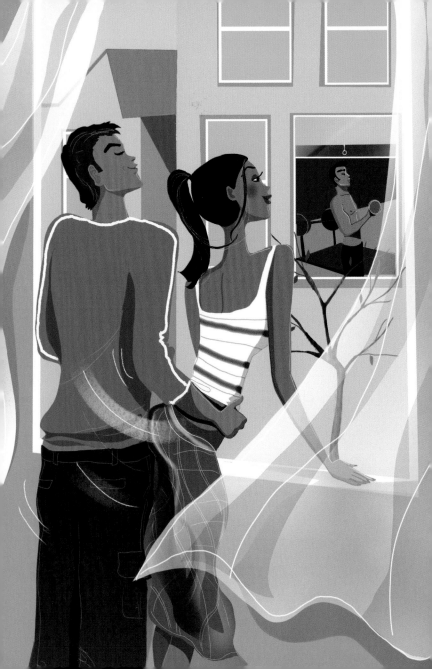

The Window

Give yourself something other than the ceiling to look at during sex—like that hot neighbor next door who never shuts their windows when they're getting undressed. You lean against a window frame. He enters you from behind.

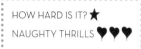

HOW HARD IS IT? ★

NAUGHTY THRILLS ♥ ♥ ♥

NICE & EASY: If you're wearing a short skirt or dress and he keeps his pants most of the way on, your neighbor won't have to know what you're doing.

WATCH OUT!!! Make sure that the window is actually closed before you start!

Backyard

Have a party under the stars—now that's romantic! You'll need an armless chaise lounge. He takes the bottom position. You straddle him and the chair. Your legs will do all the real work—he can just sit back and watch the light show.

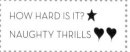

HOW HARD IS IT? ★

NAUGHTY THRILLS ♥ ♥

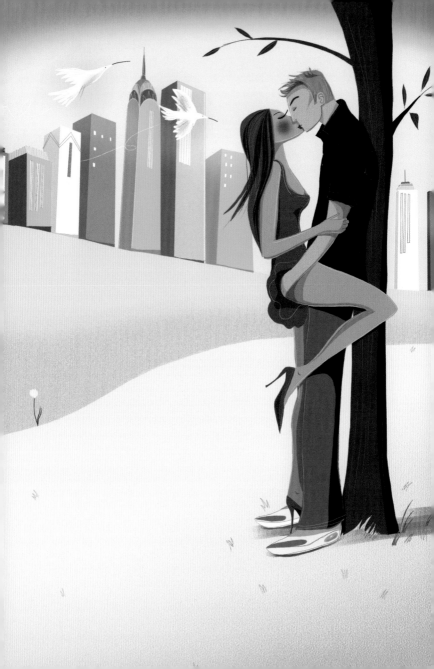

Outdoors

Save the candles, soft music and champagne for cold, windy days. When it's warm enough outside to get naked and not worry about getting frostbite on the worst places in the world to get frostbite, then a romp in the outdoors is just the thing to heat up your sex life and work on your tan at the same time. Keep these three tips in mind when getting down in the wilderness.

1. Creepy crawlers are no better to have sex with than just plain creeps. Either stay high above them by using a tree to get vertical or lay down a blanket or beach towel as a barrier to keep the pests away (if only that would work at a nightclub!).

2. Rolled up sweatshirts and big sweaters make ideal pillows and padding so the person on the ground doesn't get the wrong kind of poke.

3. Use your environment to titillate your senses. If you're at the beach, trickle sand or water over each other's naked bodies, or just enjoy the hot rays of sun and cooling breeze across areas that don't usually see the light of day.

Picnic Feast

Make sure your next outdoor feast is yummy. Pack some juicy fruit, a soft blanket and some bug-repelling candles and matches. Take the fruit and squeeze

> HOW HARD IS IT? ★
> NAUGHTY THRILLS ♥♥

the juice just below his navel and slowly lick it off, then ask him to do the same to you. Get into 69 and continue your feast.

EXTRA NAUGHTY: Gently rub the area just behind his testicles at the moment he's about to climax.

Under the Blanket

If you want to try the outdoor thing but are too nervous about being caught, or just too shy to get naked in even semi-public, pack a picnic blanket. Use the basket as your shield (hey, nothing going on here, just two people out having a picnic, something people do every day all over the world, right?). Then fold the blanket over your bodies as you slip

> HOW HARD IS IT? ★
> NAUGHTY THRILLS ♥♥

into the spoon position. It's one of the least obvious moves, and the cozy cuddling will help soothe your nervousness.

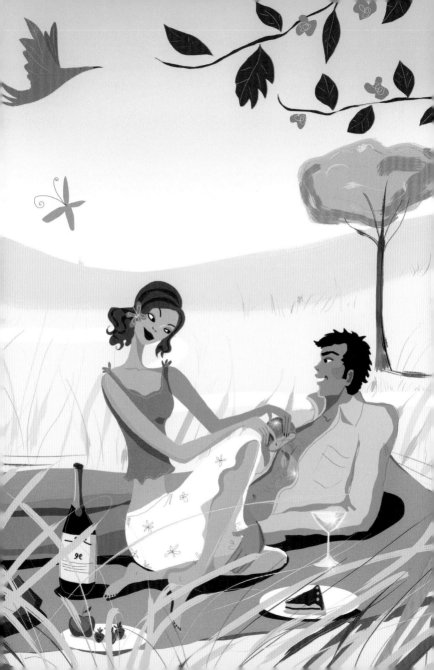

From Behind

Get into an all-fours doggy position, kneeling on the bed as he comes in from behind. Instead of holding your back flat, tilt your shoulders

HOW HARD IS IT? ★ ★ ★

NAUGHTY THRILLS ♥ ♥

downward with your forearms flat on the bed in front of you. The natural curve in your back from this variation will do all the work—expanding or contracting your

vaginal wall so you can check how deep he goes. If you arch your back into a small hump, it will shorten your vagina and shift the stimulation down a notch; drop it down and you'll feel the deeper, more intense thrusting action. Plus, he'll get strong yowzas to the head of his penis, the most sensitive part.

NICE & EASY: If you don't like him to go deep, he should start doing a hula with his hips so his pelvic bones don't push into your derrière.

Lie on your stomach. He straddles you and, to add some fanfare to his grand entrance, he holds your bottom deliciously up, so your belly presses into the mattress. He

HOW HARD IS IT? ★ ★

NAUGHTY THRILLS ♥ ♥

slips into you and leans on his forearms for support. Once he's inside of you, bring your legs together and squeeze slowly and gently. It will be like giving both of your nether regions a massage.

NICE & EASY: If you can't get the right angle, slide a big pillow under your lower body so that you're sloped in the right direction.

EXTRA NAUGHTY: He's so close to your ear that he should take advantage by having a mid-play nibble or whispering sweet, nasty nothings to you.

For some doggy action that gives you both an extra hand, have him stand on the floor beside the bed while you get on all fours at the edge of the bed. Once you start

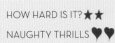

HOW HARD IS IT? ★ ★

NAUGHTY THRILLS ♥ ♥

rockin' and rollin', he should let his free hands roam over your bottom and reach around to play with your knob and up to your breasts for a quick grope.

If you're ready for your booty close-up, you can bend over the side of the bed so your stomach and breasts are pressed against the mattress and your feet are on the floor, legs spread comfortably. As he sneaks in from the back, he lifts your legs from just above the knees, holds them apart and thrusts. He gets a full rear-end view as well as getting to go in deep and hard.

HOW HARD IS IT? ★ ★

NAUGHTY THRILLS ♥

EXTRA NAUGHTY: By sliding in at an upward angle, he will knock, knock, knock against your G-spot door.

HOW HARD IS IT? ★ ★

NAUGHTY THRILLS ♥ ♥

Lie facedown across the bed with your head and upper half off the side. Put your hands on the floor to lift and lower your head. He slips between your legs so he is entering you from behind with his legs inside of your legs.

NICE & EASY: Keep it to mini-thrusts that tickle the attention-seeking first few inches of your love boat.

WATCH OUT!!! The blood is going to go straight to your head in this position, which can be a great pleasure rush, or a headache.

Benchwarmers

Parks are the next best thing to the great outdoors if your sex is in the city. But getting caught in a compromising position by nosy children isn't sexy. These easy-access

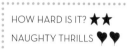

HOW HARD IS IT? ★★
NAUGHTY THRILLS ♥♥

maneuvers let you do the deed discreetly and fully clothed on a park bench. You should come prepared by wearing a long, preferably floaty, skirt and no underwear. He sits on the bench with his legs together, holding his poker straight up. You straddle his lap with your back to him and slide up and down on his tool.

NICE & EASY: He can use his hands to give your booty a boost.

WATCH OUT!!! Beware of toe-pecking pigeons.

Benchwarmer 2

Try a tantric slant on the previous benchwarmer. You sit across his lap,

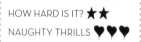

HOW HARD IS IT? ★★
NAUGHTY THRILLS ♥♥♥

your thighs at right angles to his. You then discreetly lift your skirt and wriggle gently until you've achieved the desired effect—him inside.

WATCH OUT!!! Too much jiggling will give the game away. Keep your moves slow and slight.

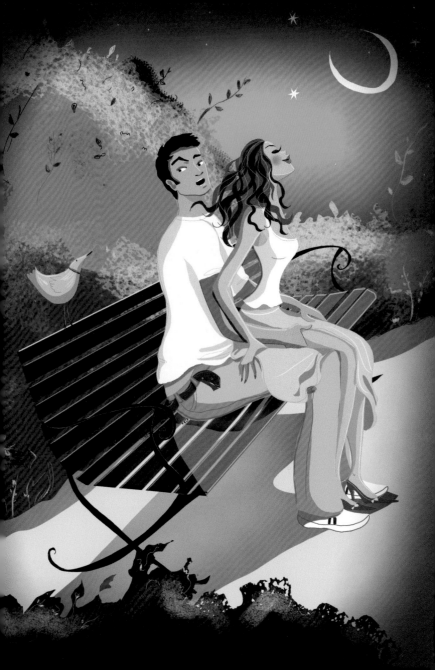

Playground Fun

Give new meaning to the word swinging by making love on a swing.
He sits on the chair and you straddle him.
To keep your balance, he can either hold
you around the waist or gently grip your
thighs. To rock and roll, move your bodies
back and forth.

HOW HARD IS IT? ★★★

NAUGHTY THRILLS ♥

More Playground Fun

Another variation of swinging sex is for you to sit on the edge, raise
your legs and put them on his shoulders while he stands in front of you.
He enters you and grabs the front of the swing. You may have to adjust
the height of the swing to get yourselves lined up. He can now move
you back and forth with the swing, so that his penis strokes in and out
with each movement. Result: a weightless
lovemaking sensation.

HOW HARD IS IT? ★★

NAUGHTY THRILLS ♥ ♥

Make Like a Sand Crab

HOW HARD IS IT? ★
NAUGHTY THRILLS ♥ ♥

Lay out your beach towel (bigger is better in this case). He sits on the towel, you climb onto his lap, and shimmy up and down his shaft.

NICE & EASY: If the beach is rush-hour crowded, you can slip a sarong over your swimsuit to hide the action. Then all you have to do is pull aside the crotch of your bottoms.

Avoiding Sandy Cracks

A "shore" thing can end up a wash in no time if you aren't careful. The gritty rub of sand in your crack can kill the romantic waves-pounding-canoodling-in-the-surf mood faster than you can say "wipe out." To avoid a sandy groin, find a quiet dune. You kneel on all fours with legs wide. He kneels on his knees, right up against your rear.

HOW HARD IS IT? ★
NAUGHTY THRILLS ♥ ♥ ♥

EXTRA NAUGHTY: You can clench your thighs together so you can feel every move he makes.

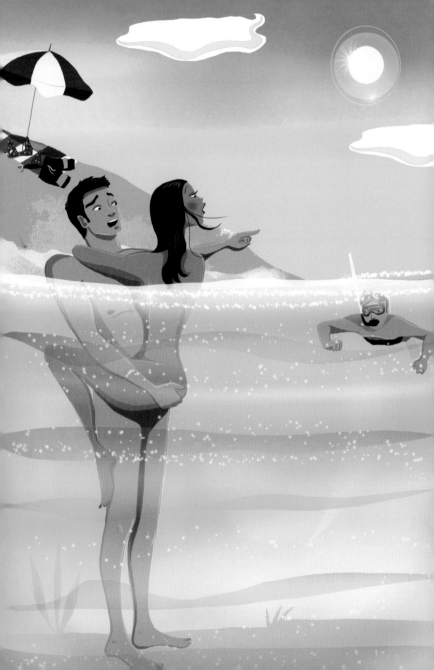

Lotion Up

To melt each other under the sun in full view of all the sun worshippers, use sand-repellent sunscreen and massage each other to bliss.

HOW HARD IS IT? ★
NAUGHTY THRILLS ♥ ♥ ♥

Skinny Dipping

Make your own waves with this splashy move. Find your own blue lagoon and get ready to dirty dance. You stand with your back facing your guy. He lifts you up by the waist, slowly angling your body—legs spreading to each side of his torso—until your crotch meets his at a 90-degree angle. To (skinny) dip, he should direct his erect member in and out of your body while holding onto you firmly.

WATCH OUT!!! This move needs privacy.

HOW HARD IS IT? ★ ★ ★
NAUGHTY THRILLS ♥

Waterfall Fun

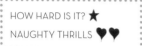

HOW HARD IS IT? ★

NAUGHTY THRILLS ♥ ♥

Using a waterfall as a screen, you stand in front and he slides in from behind. The water will cascade over your bodies like 100 caressing fingers and shield your fun and games from prying eyes at the same time.

Into the Woods

The woods are full of thorny pinecones, stinging nettles, fire ants and so much more that's risky to bare butts. Instead of thrashing around on the ground, this yoga-like move keeps all your nakedness and delicate parts away from poking, scratching or burrowing. To get into position, you bend over and touch

HOW HARD IS IT? ★

NAUGHTY THRILLS ♥ ♥

your knees. He stands with his knees bent and legs shoulder-width apart for balance, and enters you from behind.

NICE & EASY: He can hold your hips so that you don't tip over and possibly snap his branch. If you keep toppling over, stand within an arm's length of a tree so you can support yourself at a 90-degree angle.

EXTRA NAUGHTY: Holding your hips also means he can push deep into you.

Another Tree-Hugging Move

HOW HARD IS IT? ★★

NAUGHTY THRILLS ♥♥

A variation to the above position begins with you leaning against the tree as before, but instead of tilting in the same direction as you, he presses his hips against yours and, holding onto your hips for balance, leans back in the opposite direction. The opposite pull of your upper bodies creates incredible tension—just be sure your friction doesn't start a forest fire.

Grassy Meadow

Languor in the grass, feel the light tickle of the blades against your skin and sink into the softness of the ground. You lie on your stomach and elbows. He lies on top of you with his weight on his arms.

NICE & EASY: You can raise your bottom slightly to increase penetration.

HOW HARD IS IT? ★

NAUGHTY THRILLS ♥♥

Hill Start

Stand on a hill, facing each other. You stand on ground that's a little more elevated than where he's standing. You then slightly twist toward the side and

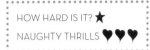

HOW HARD IS IT? ★

NAUGHTY THRILLS ♥ ♥ ♥

place one leg a few steps up the incline to give him easy entry. Once he's inside of you, you can hold onto him by grasping him around the lower waist while he keeps you steady by gently holding your hips.

NICE & EASY: Thrust-wise, it's best if he just swings his hips—anything more forceful can throw you both off balance.

Car-ma Sutra

A classic car-ma pose is for you to sit on the hood and wrap your legs around his waist as he stands, leaning back and supporting yourself with your arms. You can control the motion by thrusting with your pelvis or pulling him toward you with your legs. You may also brace your feet on the car bumper on either side of him for better leverage.

NICE & EASY: Warm the engine up a bit first so the hood isn't booty-freezing cold.

EXTRA NAUGHTY: Let the car ride you to orgasm—shake enough so it gets rocking and then go with its move to get into the groove.

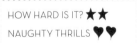

HOW HARD IS IT? ★ ★

NAUGHTY THRILLS ♥ ♥

WATCH OUT: Check that the car alarm has been turned off, or your spring fling is going to turn into a spectator sport.

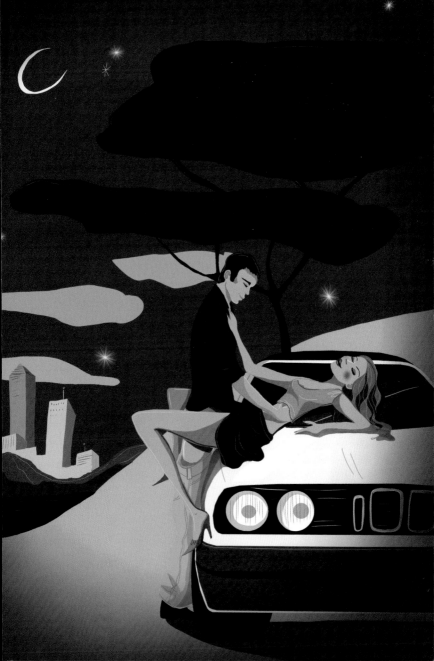

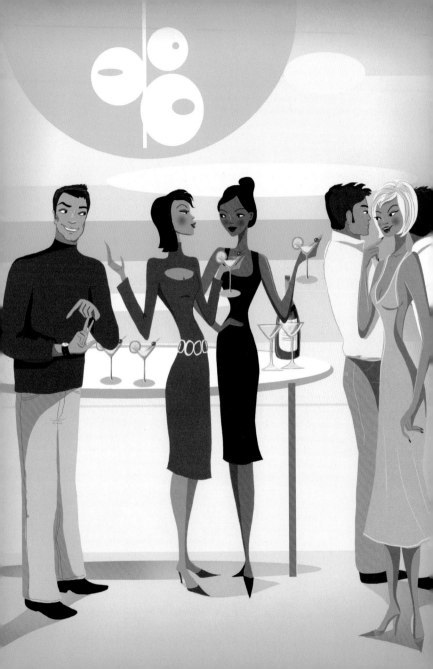

In Public

Why is public sex so incredibly exciting? Simple biology. The fear of getting caught causes rapid production of adrenaline, the sexy pick-me-up you manufacture when you're aroused. In short, you're scaring yourself into an awesome orgasm. Keep these five tips in mind for pulling off sex in public without a hitch.

1. Dress for speed. Wear an easy-to-lift dress or skirt and skip the pantyhose and underwear. Nothing below his belt should require more than one button.

2. Have a starting plan. Use a special code phrase or gesture that means "let's do it now" so you can slip out discreetly.

3. Forget foreplay. The thrill you get from doing it somewhere you shouldn't (along with a quick squirt from the tiny lube packet hidden in his wallet) will equal at least one hour of foreplay.

4. Be selfish. This is the wrong place to work on your relationship and there is no time to worry about his feelings. Do whatever it takes to get yourself off and assume he is doing the same.

5. Have a stopping plan. Getting caught might be half the fun, but be ready to stop the fun and vacate the location as quickly as possible if someone walks in on you.

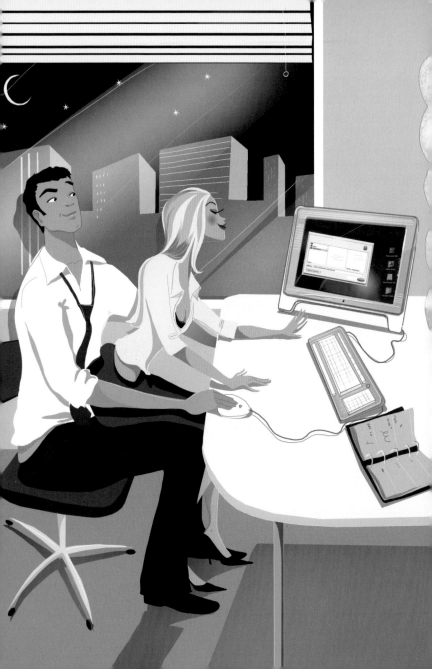

At the Office 1

Dive under the desk—your bodies will probably fit best at an angle. The person visiting the cubicle owner should be on the bottom so that they are least visible (if there is room, they should scrunch up their legs as much as possible). The owner of the cubicle then dives under the desk so that all that is visible is their legs, which will (hopefully, sort of, let's face it you're not fooling anyone) look like they are searching for something.

NICE & EASY: Put a stack of files on the floor beside the desk so if anyone pops their head in, you can stand up and say, "Oops, I dropped all my folders!" Bonus: You can use the folders to cover up anything hanging out that shouldn't be.

At the Office 2

If your office is private, use a chair without wheels and flick on the computer monitor for sexy mood lighting. He sits and you perch on his lap. Rest your elbows on the desk for support and resist the urge to check your emails.

EXTRA NAUGHTY 1: Log onto a porn site first (www.nerve.com is classy, and it's unlikely to raise red flags if your log-on action is monitored).

EXTRA NAUGHTY 2: Give yourself an instant promotion and move the action to your boss's office (giving yourself something to smile about during those boring staff meetings).

In the Conference Room

He lifts you onto the table. You scoot to the edge and lie back. He stands at the edge, lifts your legs into the air and holds them together in front of you. This will keep the friction up and keep your hands busy, so no incriminating fingerprints are left on the table.

NICE & EASY: Keep one eye on the door.

WATCH OUT!!! Clean up after you, people—make sure no used condoms have ended up in a dark corner.

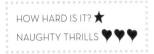

HOW HARD IS IT? ★

NAUGHTY THRILLS ♥ ♥ ♥

At a Boring Party

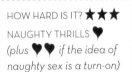

HOW HARD IS IT? ★ ★ ★

NAUGHTY THRILLS ♥

(plus ♥ ♥ if the idea of naughty sex is a turn-on)

Slip into the coat closet. It'll be a tight fit so you'll want a move that doesn't require a course in acrobatics. Unfortunately, the male and female physiques rarely match up in a way that makes this feasible. To get them in line, he will need to brace himself against the two walls penning you in—his feet flat on the floor pushing into the wall in front of him and, standing so he is in a slight squat position, his back pushing into the opposite wall. His legs should be hip-width apart. You stand with your legs straddling his thighs, then you sit in his hands as he lifts you up, using the two walls for stability. Wrap your legs around him and bounce in place.

NICE & EASY: It helps if you can stand on a couple of old phone books.

WATCH OUT!!! Don't use a door as one of your walls—it could unexpectedly pop open under the pressure.

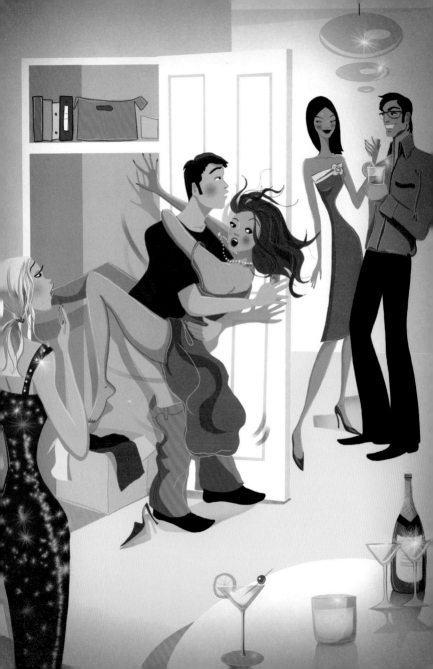

At a Restaurant

You can have a sex apéritif right at your table by taking turns giving each other hand jobs. Request a banquette or a table that has a long cloth (both found

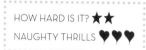

HOW HARD IS IT? ★★

NAUGHTY THRILLS ♥ ♥ ♥

in restaurants with more than one star). At the banquette, instead of sitting side-by-side (where your jerky arms will be a dead giveaway that you're lighting your own fire and the awkward angle can lead to arm cramps), take turns pretending to be the more-in-love partner who sits half-facing the object of their affection. Make sure whoever is doing the dirty work is seated so that the hand they usually work with is on the side closest to their partner. If you're at a table, then sit at adjacent corners (same rules apply regarding arm location). Use your napkin as a drop cloth and for soaking up any stray juices. Bon appétit!

NICE & EASY: Do the restaurant staff a favor and take the napkin home with you.

WATCH OUT!!! Chairs with armrests block access.

Take a Cab

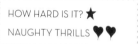

HOW HARD IS IT? ★

NAUGHTY THRILLS ♥ ♥

If you are hailing a taxi, don't worry about the driver when feeding each other's meters—they've seen a lot worse. Fall back into the seat in a close embrace, then you straddle him and undo his fly. The overall effect should be of a couple of hot and horny vacationers engaging in some passionate necking.

NICE & EASY: You should slip into a skirt to conceal the action.

WATCH OUT!!! Make sure you keep track of the miles so you reach home base by the time you get to your destination.

At a Sporting Event

Head to the back of the crowded, rowdy fan section where everyone is too obsessed with the game to notice your bumps and grinds. He quietly unzips, then stands behind you and holds you in a big hug. With his arms wrapped around your chest for balance, he can bend his knees slightly so that his pelvis is below yours. You should arch your back, prop one foot on the back of the seat in front of you, and stand with your legs apart so you're ready to have the ball passed to you.

NICE & EASY: You can use the roar of the crowd to camouflage your own roars.

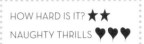

HOW HARD IS IT? ★★

NAUGHTY THRILLS ♥ ♥ ♥

WATCH OUT!!! You need to be in a skirt with a jacket tied around your waist or you'll be providing more entertainment to the crowd than the cheerleaders.

Shop 'Til You Drop

There's nothing better to boost your mood than a little shopping therapy. To counter the boredom for your man, slip into a changing room together—you can say you

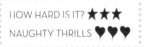

HOW HARD IS IT? ★★★

NAUGHTY THRILLS ♥ ♥ ♥

want him to check out your outfit. Since changing room walls are often flimsy, which means they could collapse mid-thrust, it's best if he sits on the bench and you sit on top facing away, legs spread and feet on the floor. Subtle bounces should get you both where you want to go.

NICE & EASY: Ideally, you'll want a retail store that is big enough for no one to be paying attention to you, but small enough that people aren't constantly streaming through the changing room.

EXTRA NAUGHTY: Try to pick a room that has a mirror opposite the bench so you can check yourselves out mid-action.

In a Public Restroom

Although wonderful for adding a little privacy to your public show, restrooms are not always so nice for other obvious reasons, so choose your location wisely. The easiest is a nightclub stall—they practically expect you to have sex there. For the best atmosphere, head for a fancy restaurant or hotel, which will probably have nice-smelling restrooms and lots of products on hand to freshen up with after. Keep in mind that the ladies' usually has more privacy and is cleaned more often than the men's room. Wherever you are, you will want to avoid bare body contact with the surrounding surfaces. He presses your back against the door of the stall as you prop your foot on the seat of the toilet or toilet paper dispenser for support. He should crouch down so his plunger is lower and angled up toward your plumbing, then slip it in and start pumping.

HOW HARD IS IT? ★★★
NAUGHTY THRILLS ♥

Join the 60 mph Club

When you are ready to drive each other wild, jump in the car and start your engines. Give each other a hand-squeezer while driving—when the driver's legs involuntarily close with pleasure, pull over and finish the trip on a quiet side street. Once parked, he gets in the passenger seat and you sit on his lap facing him with your knees pushed against your chest and your feet on the seat. You won't be able to get much movement, so you should squeeze your thighs to press the horn on your love accessories.

HOW HARD IS IT? ★★
NAUGHTY THRILLS ♥

NICE & EASY: You can also try facing away from him with your feet on the car floor.

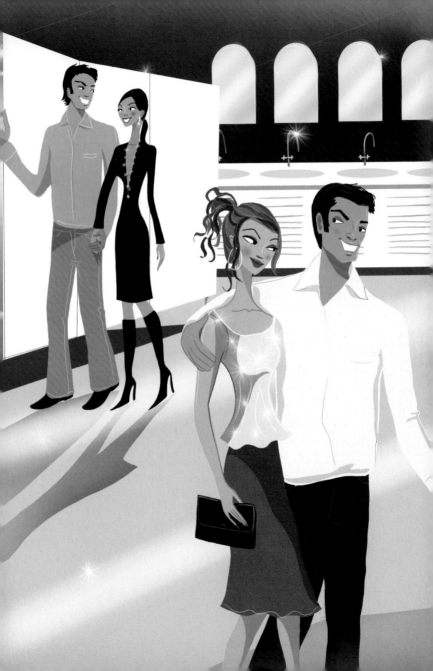

Girl On Top

Lie him back on the bed, face him and lower yourself onto his passion crank in a kneeling position. Keeping your knees on the bed, hook your feet over the inside of his legs (aim for his knees). Grabbing the sheets on either side of his head, squeeze your booty, tilt your pelvis upwards and move in small, tight motions. As long as you hold on tight, you can ride him wild until you are both lassoed by orgasms.

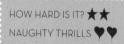

HOW HARD IS IT? ★ ★
NAUGHTY THRILLS ♥ ♥

NICE & EASY: You should ride his body high so his pubic bone rubs against your joy button.

He lies flat on his back with his legs straight out and spread slightly. Standing with your feet flat by his sides, you squat over his hips so

HOW HARD IS IT? ★ ★ ★
NAUGHTY THRILLS ♥ ♥ ♥

you're facing his feet. As you guide his penis inside, give it a few quick squeezes as a taste of what's to come. Sit on his lower abdomen with your legs bent and

lean forward, bracing yourself with your hands on his knees, and start moving up and down.

NICE & EASY: He reaches both hands around your waist and playfully squeezes your nipples and massages your swollen clitoris.

EXTRA NAUGHTY: Instead of the usual follow-the-bouncing-ball up and down movements, try lateral jerks to really hit your hot zones. Or wiggle your hips in a circular motion to caress every inch of your vagina with his penis.

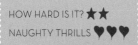
Guys are visual creatures—he sees a naked female and he stands right to attention. So squatting over him, looking straight at him, with your feet flat on either side and playing with yourself will tweak his interest rapidly. He sees breasts, vagina, your hands playing with said breasts and vagina—what's not to love?

NICE & EASY: Your hands should stray down to his power tool to make sure it's turned on.

EXTRA NAUGHTY: You can tease him by letting him enter just a fraction, then lifting yourself tantalizingly higher.

Teasing him while you are on top is a great way to win the sack race. Have him lie on his back while you climb on top and straddle him. Then lower yourself onto his penis, but go no further than the very tip

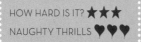
of the glans. Then back away by lifting yourself up. Repeat nine times. On the tenth, lower yourself all the way down on his penis, letting it thrust fully into your vagi-port. Before he can get comfortably berthed, pull yourself back up and begin your next set of attack and retreat, but this time counting eight shallow thrusts and two deep ones, followed by seven shallow and three deep, and so on. By the time you reach ten deep thrusts, you'll have lost count!

NICE & EASY: If you don't have thigh muscles of steel, you can try leaning forward over him and using your abdominal muscles to lift your pelvis up and down until you collapse in delight.

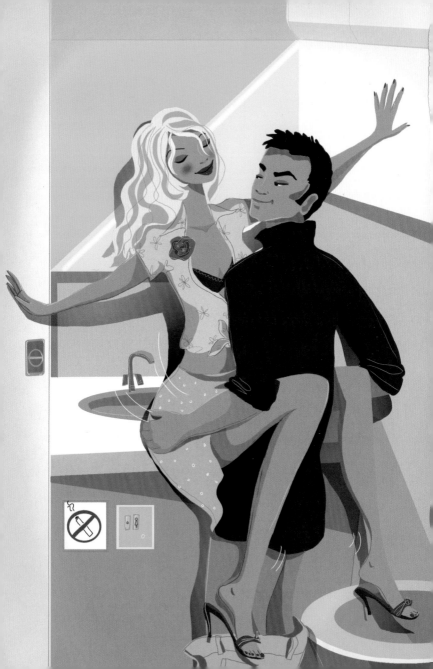

Join the Mile High Club

When you're flying, why not get your membership in the Mile High Club? You should meet at an agreed-upon toilet that is not visible from the galleys where flight attendants may be hanging out. Once you are both inside, he should sit on the closed toilet seat and you sit on his lap facing away from him. This way, neither of you will be too close to the ceiling, risking a concussion if it is a bumpy ride.

HOW HARD IS IT? ★ ★ ★
NAUGHTY THRILLS ♥ ♥

NICE & EASY: Stand up and lean over the sink so you can watch yourselves in the mirror (this beats flying first class every time).

EXTRA NAUGHTY: Turn around and perch yourself on the edge of the sink with him standing between your legs. You should keep your hands pressed against the opposite wall and door to prevent yourself from slipping and possibly crash landing on his li'l pilot.

WATCH OUT!!! It's illegal to have sex in an airplane bathroom—so deny it in the unlikely event that you are asked. Tell the flight attendant or other passengers that one of you was ill and the other was playing nurse.

Junior Membership in the Club

If lavatory sex leaves you cold, you can still join the club with some discreetly done moves in your seats. It will be easiest if you can get an exit row since you will need every bit of space. First, snag a couple of blankets, turn off the overhead light and raise the armrest. Then it's amazingly easy to hide a hand job under one of those little airplane blankets. And if you're really sneaky, you can rest your head on your partner's lap and just happen to have oral sex. But try not to let your head bob up and down (unless there's turbulence).

HOW HARD IS IT? ★ ★

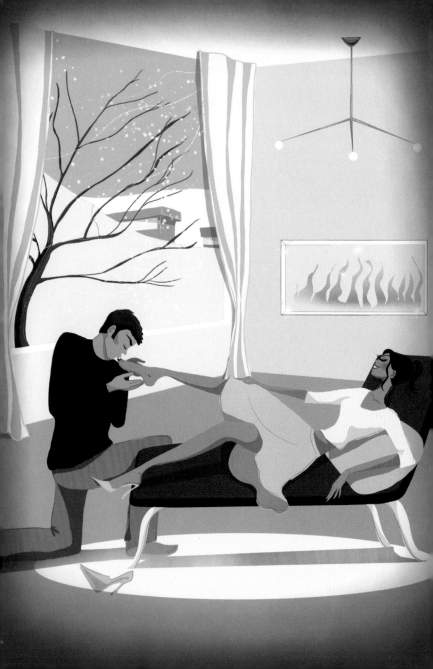

Vacations and Holidays

Time off work is the ultimate postmodern aphrodisiac. A day away from the daily grind is the perfect time for some pleasurable bump and grind. And with all that free time between 9 and 5, you'll have no excuse for making due with a quickie. Turn off your Blackberry, turn on your out-of-office autoreply, and have him get to work filling up your inbox.

If you didn't burn all his jet fuel on the getaway flight (turn back one page if you missed that trick!), you're going to want to start your vacation off right with some packing and unpacking. But don't stay in your room the whole time, hotels and resorts offer an array of hot spots for vacation relations.

At the end of the year, when you get time off work for the holidays, don't spend it all waiting in line to sit on Santa's lap (unless you're into that kind of thing). Try turning your X-mas break into twelve days of XXX-giving (and receiving).

Lazy Day Sex

When relaxing on a vacation, you barely want to move, let alone pump up the action. Slip into a hammock so that he's on bottom and you're lying flat on top. He can wrap his arms around you and you can do the same with your legs around him. Very slowly sway your way to a sweet, slow climax.

HOW HARD IS IT? ★

NAUGHTY THRILLS ♥

Swimming Lessons

Quiet times at the hotel pool late at night and early in the morning offer an opportunity for a first class upgrade to your hotel stay. Have him give you a fake swimming lesson. Slip on a pair of inflatable armbands, which allow you to float on your back, while he stands at your side, cradling you in his arms. You let your inside arm slip beneath the waves and into his suit. He does the same to you. Practice this "stroke" together until the water gets too heated.

HOW HARD IS IT? ★ ★

NAUGHTY THRILLS ♥ ♥ ♥

Create Your Own Pleasure Island

Squeeze into an extra-large floating ring facing each other. This way you won't have to worry about floating away from each other in the middle of your water games. People nearby will just think you're bobbing in place.

HOW HARD IS IT? ★

NAUGHTY THRILLS ♥ ♥ ♥

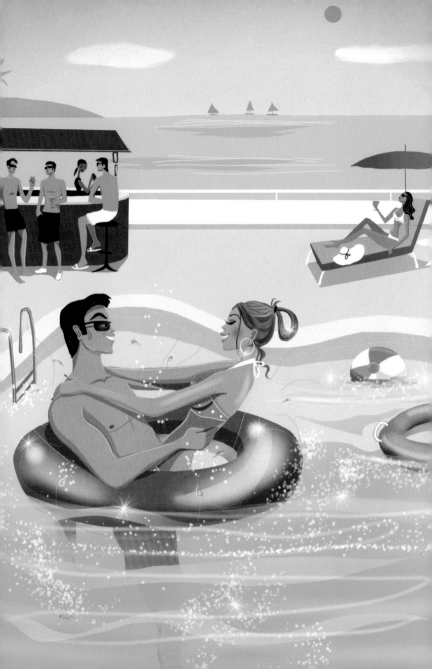

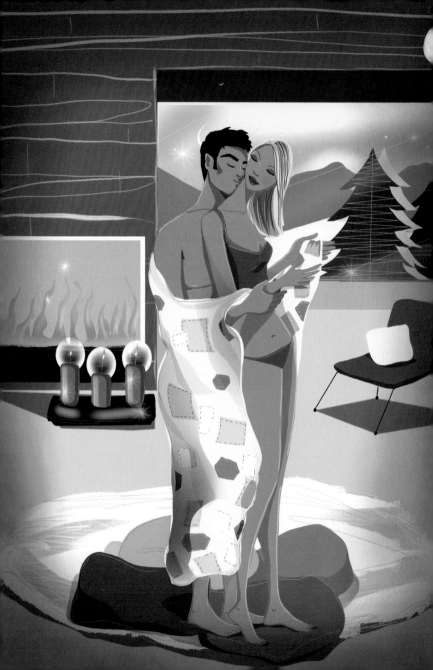

Cold Weather Cuddling

Looking for a way to generate enough heat to melt the snow off the roof of your alpine lodge? You don't need to have sex to have a whole-body sexual experience (don't rub your eyes, you did read that correctly). This all-over cozy body cuddle might or might not lead to intercourse—it's your call. But either way, it will leave you feeling totally connected to your partner. You can do it standing up, on a rug by the fire or in the bed, though to devote some real snuggle time to each other, begin in bed and stay that way.

Lying down, start in a spooning position with both of you on the same side, facing in the same direction. Close your eyes and relax, letting all the tension ooze out of your bodies. Try to breathe in sync. Once your breathing is matched, continue for five minutes.

NICE & EASY: This is a great way to start your day.

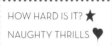

HOW HARD IS IT? ★

NAUGHTY THRILLS ♥

EXTRA NAUGHTY: He can start your engine by reaching around and playing squeeze the fruit with your breasts or hunt the pea in your love garden.

The "HOT" Tub

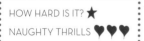

HOW HARD IS IT? ★

NAUGHTY THRILLS ♥ ♥ ♥

The cold mountain air will not be enough to put the frostbite on this action. He keeps his snorkeller out of water as he sits on the edge of a hot tub with his legs in the water. Turn the jets on high. You sit or kneel between his legs on the ledge in the water so you get a steady blast of hot bubbles to your rub-a-dub. While your lower half is pulsating, you give his diver a little mouth resuscitation.

WATCH OUT!!! Hot water can cause blood vessels to dilate, turning his timber into a limp twig.

Standing

You stand facing your partner with your left foot turned out and your right foot forward. His legs should be slightly bent, spaced about

HOW HARD IS IT? ★ ★ ★

NAUGHTY THRILLS ♥ ♥

three feet apart. With your arms on his shoulders and his arms around your lower back, you slowly pull your right leg up and prop your right foot on his left shoulder. After he sinks his putt, you ease into a vertical split by sliding your calf as far up his left shoulder as you comfortably can.

WATCH OUT!!! While you don't have to have been a former gymnast to make the groove with this move, you should be able to touch your toes without bending your knees.

This move mimics the standing forward bend (pada hasthasana) in yoga, but packs more of an erotic punch. You bend forward with your legs slightly spread and your arms either hanging loose in front of you (you can rest them on a low chair if you need the extra balance). He moves in from behind, pulling himself as close to you as possible while holding onto your body for sheer delight.

HOW HARD IS IT? ★ - ★ ★

NAUGHTY THRILLS ♥ ♥

EXTRA NAUGHTY: Instead of moving in and out, grind your behind in circles.

You get on all fours on the floor, and he enters you from behind. He then wraps his arms around your thighs as he stands up (he should look as if he's pushing a wheelbarrow).

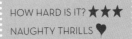

NICE & EASY: Walk around on your hands, with him thrusting as you go.

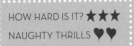

Start with him sitting on a chair. Facing him, lower yourself onto his erect penis until you're sitting on his lap. While you wrap your arms and legs tightly around him, he cradles your lower back and bottom while he slowly stands up.

NICE & EASY: Propping your back up against a wall for support or resting your rear end on a table will make this move easier for him.

EXTRA NAUGHTY: If he's been working on his guns at the gym, he should be strong enough to lift you up and down on his penis.

With him standing in front of you like a stairway to heaven, you can walk your way to the orgasmic stratosphere with this move. You lie naked on the edge of

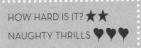

the bed with your feet on the floor. He stands on the floor and enters you. As he begins thrusting, you raise your legs and you "walk the wall," climbing his chest by putting one foot in front of the other. You climb up and down "the wall" until you find the angle of penetration you like best.

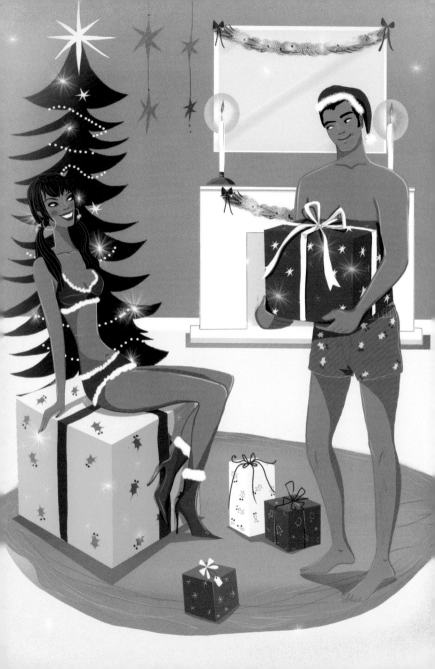

12 Days of XXX-mas

Add the following seasonal twist to these 12 naughty tricks and you'll enter the new year singing "falalalalalaaaaa!"

1ST DAY: Take him out gift shopping and do something that guarantees you'll end up on Santa's naughty list this year. *See Shopping, page 75*

2ND DAY: Go to a cut-your-own tree farm and arrive at dusk so that no one will see you as you chop down his tree. *See Woods, page 64*

3RD DAY: At your office holiday party, skip Secret Santa and show him a few secrets Santa doesn't know. *See Conference Room, page 72*

4TH DAY: Ask him to help you hang the stockings by the chimney with care. Then roast his chestnuts near the open fire. *See Fuzzy Feeling, page 37*

5TH DAY: Make a date with him to bake holiday cookies, then make some cookie nookie for yourselves. *See Kitchen Counter, page 38*

6TH DAY: Let the twinkling lights from the tree turn the darkened room into your own personal strip club. *See Private Dancer, page 104*

7TH DAY: Try out the high-tech features on the new camcorder you bought to capture the holiday memories. Just don't send Grandma the wrong DVD! *See Porn Star, page 101*

8TH DAY: Drive around admiring the festive light displays. Then park and put on a flashy display of your own. *See 60 mph Club, page 76*

9TH DAY: Join a group of carolers spreading some seasonal joy. But after a few houses, make some joy yourself. *See Bench Warmer, page 58*

10TH DAY: Ditch the neighbor's lame party and set your date's yule log on fire. *See At a Boring Party, page 72*

11TH DAY: Tease him by sucking a candy cane. Before its stripes are gone, his sugar stick will be as hard as candy. *See Oral Sex on Him, pages 14-15.*

12TH DAY: Remember the great toys you got as a kid? Buy each other a grown-up toy and see how much fun you can have. *See Toys, pages 117-21.*

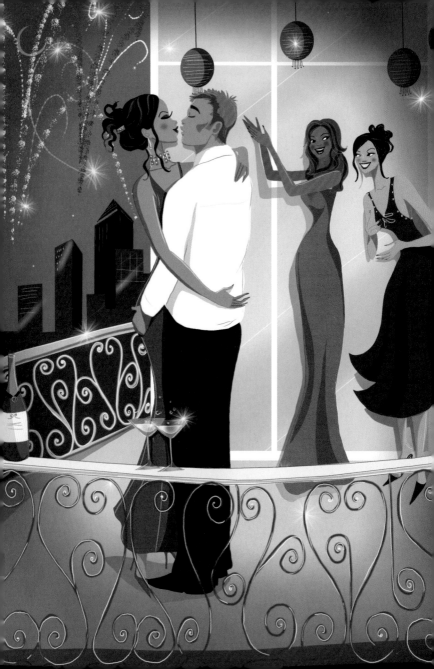

Pop Your Cork Early

New Year's Eve sex is often a messy, shoddy, unsatisfactory affair. You're both too tired and champagne-fueled to do anything more than make a few half-hearted gropes before collapsing mid-play. This is why it makes sense to have a quick fix before you hit the party circuit. He lifts you up onto a waist-high surface, you open your legs wide and in he goes. He thrusts in and out from the front, which will rub against your G-spot. Result: You create mega-heat in a minimal amount of time and your lipstick won't even get mussed.

WATCH OUT!!! Because of the angle, the head of his penis will be rubbing your inner body in such a way that he may leave the party early. If he's about to pop his cork, he should pull out for a second, recover and begin again.

HOW HARD IS IT? ★★

NAUGHTY THRILLS ♥ ♥

Easy Lay

Tradition has it to see the old year out with a bonk. Fine, if you were actually in any condition to operate body parts. Since you're not, go for something effortless. Start in missionary and flip onto your sides—now you'll barely need to move at all and best of all, you can fall asleep in exactly the same position you made love in.

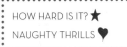

HOW HARD IS IT? ★

NAUGHTY THRILLS ♥

NICE & EASY: You can wrap one leg around him for deeper penetration and to hold him closer, creating even more of a loving connection.

EXTRA NAUGHTY: If he moves his body slightly away from yours, he will be able to penetrate deeper. Although this may be something he wants to save for when you wake up in position the following morning.

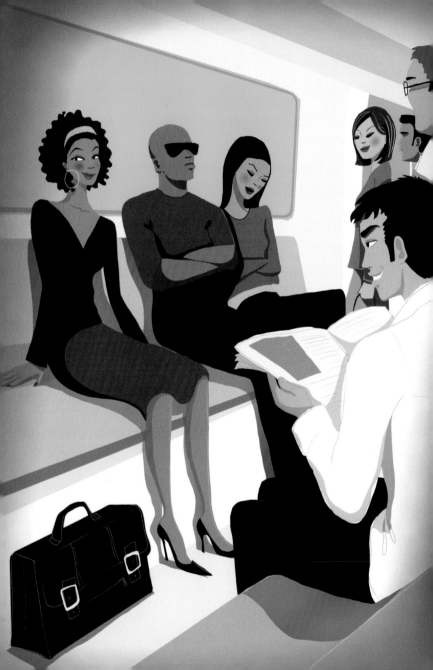

7

Fantasy

He's always known you were a nice girl. And by now you've shown him that you can also be naughty in the bedroom...and beyond! But wherever and whichever way you have been doing it, your prime time show has always starred the same two characters. It's time to boost your ratings by changing some roles without changing the leading man or his star actress.

Maybe you think cowboys are hot. Just because he can't wrastle a steer doesn't mean you can't ride him like a bronco. Or perhaps the thought of you dressed in a French maid outfit gives him ideas of waxing something other than the furniture. Pretend you are the script writers and let your imaginations create one blockbuster sexy scene after another.

Buckin' Bronco

He sits on the bed with his legs extended and knees bent. You sit in his lap and lower yourself onto his erect penis with your feet flat on the bed. You then lean back with your hands on the bed for support.

EXTRA NAUGHTY 1: You straddle his lap with your knees on the floor, and then lean into a backbend (being careful not to strain your lower back).

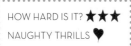

HOW HARD IS IT? ★ ★ ★

NAUGHTY THRILLS ♥

EXTRA NAUGHTY 2: You then lean back fully to rest the top of your head on the bed and reach back with your hands until they grasp his feet.

Cinderella and Prince Charming

He sweeps you off your feet and treats you to an orgasmic oral ball that a princess like you deserves. He gives it a royal twist by lifting your thigh onto his shoulders and raising your lower body off the bed so you are

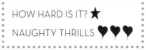

HOW HARD IS IT? ★

NAUGHTY THRILLS ♥ ♥ ♥

essentially upside down. This will completely open you up to receive his majestic pleasure.

EXTRA NAUGHTY: He can hum while he is down there. It will create a buzz on your lower lips that works exactly like a vibrator.

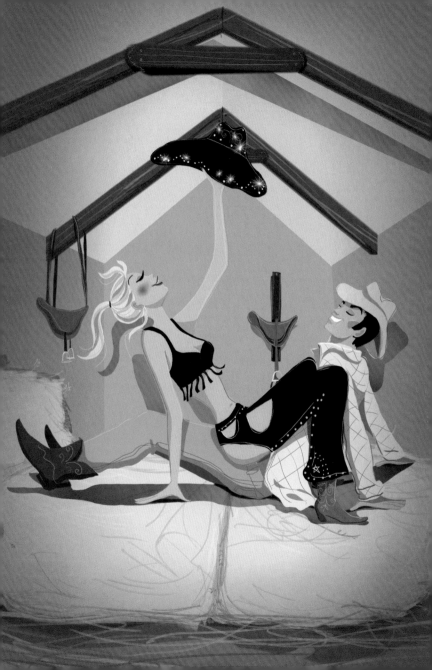

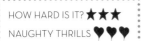

Master and Maid

HOW HARD IS IT? ★ ★ ★

NAUGHTY THRILLS ♥ ♥ ♥

He wears a stylish tuxedo with a bow tie around his neck. You dress in a frilly French maid's outfit. You untie his tie, and he returns the favor by tying your hands together and then your feet together. Once he has you bound, he carries you to a soft surface and sets you up on your elbows and knees. He comes in from behind to ravish you mercilessly.

Dominatrix

You dress in leather and sport a riding crop, while he's in briefs. You then order him to lie parallel to you and match your own self-love technique, mano-a-mano. He must reach between your legs with the same hand you usually use to please yourself. You put your gloved hand over his and bark directions at him, all the while lightly flicking your riding crop against his bottom. He must continue until you tell him to stop.

NICE & EASY: He should lubricate his finger with your juices.

EXTRA NAUGHTY: He has to get into whatever position you pick.

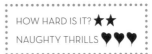

HOW HARD IS IT? ★ ★

NAUGHTY THRILLS ♥ ♥ ♥

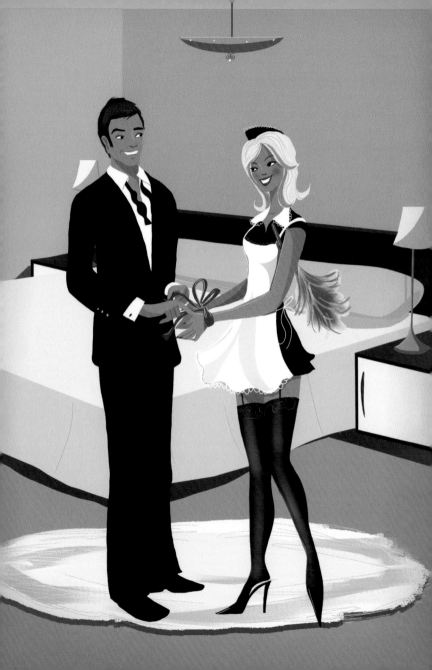

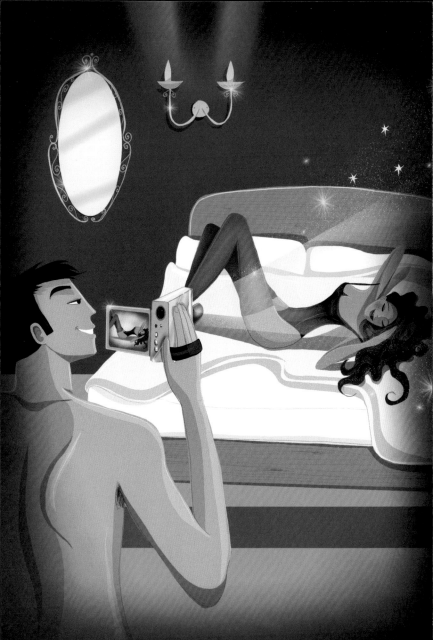

Porn Star

Filming your own sex video can make you feel as hot as the hottest porn star. And as an added bonus, once you get famous, you'll be able to buy copies of your own movie off the Internet. But if you are going to make love like a porn star, then you will want to follow these lessons from top skin flicks.

1. DITCH THE BRIGHT, OVERHEAD LIGHTING

It's unflattering, making you look like a past-your-prime porn star. Instead, use low light at a low height to create romantic shadows that give your body a sensuous edge.

2. KEEP YOUR SHIRT ON

Usually you get naked when you have sex. Don't. Get started doing oral sex before the clothes hit the floor and leave as much sexy lingerie on as possible during intercourse.

3. USE YOUR HEAD

The camera isn't going to capture you wagging your tongue or cranking your jaw until it is ready to drop off, so move your entire noggin during mouth sex.

4. SAVOR THE FEELING

He penetrates slowly, then withdraws completely, waits a second and then starts over. This will allow the tension to build and looks great on film since he is keeping everything out in the open!

5. BOUNCE

This is your one chance to shine, so it's no time to let him steal the scene. Climb on top and move your body up and down, front and back, side to side. Plus, this will up the friction factor—giddy-up and away!

6. DON'T FINISH WHERE YOU STARTED

Three minutes is about as long as you'll see any "actor" in the same position—they move around to keep things interesting.

Sitting

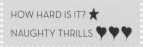

HOW HARD IS IT? ★
NAUGHTY THRILLS ♥♥♥

Instead of letting him sit all the way down on the bed, have him get on his knees and sit back so that his backside is resting on his ankles. This will elevate and push forward your target. Climb on top facing him—squat down so he slides inside and do a pelvic grind.

EXTRA NAUGHTY: You can shimmy up and down until you find the angle that makes his hammer nail your pleasure nut.

He parks himself in an armless chair that's narrow enough for you to comfortably straddle. You then hop on his pogo stick and bounce up and down to your heart's content.

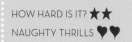

HOW HARD IS IT? ★★
NAUGHTY THRILLS ♥♥

EXTRA NAUGHTY: He should keep his feet together and tilt his hips upward—this angling gives you a good grinding surface to work against.

This move is a bit of a workout but worth the burn. He sits with his hands behind him for support, his legs splayed open, knees slightly bent. While keeping your hands on the surface for support, face him, straddle his lap, and rest your right leg on his right shoulder and your left leg on his left shoulder. The angle of his dangle will bring on deep G-spot orgasms.

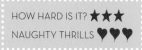

HOW HARD IS IT? ★★★
NAUGHTY THRILLS ♥♥♥

This is a sit-down move for when the urge strikes you at your desk or even after a romantic meal. He relaxes back against the chair, legs spread comfortably, feet on the floor. You straddle his lap with your back to him, your body inside his legs, arms stretched out in front of you so they reach the desk/tabletop and your legs close together. He holds your hips tightly to his lap with your feet suspended in the air. He'll be able to tease every inch of your vagina with deep up-and-down motions.

HOW HARD IS IT? ★★
NAUGHTY THRILLS ♥ ♥ ♥

EXTRA NAUGHTY: To send you into orgasmic overdrive, he can shift gears by using circular strokes.

Reconnect with each other by sitting in the center of your bed facing each other. You wrap your legs comfortably around his body so you're sitting on his thighs. Place your right hand at the back of his neck and your left hand at the base of his spine; he should mirror you. When he cranks his shaft in you, he should be giving your love bell a ring-a-ding-ling at the same time. Rock together slowly, rubbing each other's backs and kissing deeply with your eyes open until you both orgasm.

HOW HARD IS IT? ★★★
NAUGHTY THRILLS ♥ ♥ ♥

NICE & EASY: Put stacks of pillows behind you so one of you can lean back if you feel the need to recline.

Private Dancer

Giving him a private lap dance is sure to please him, and may even get you twenty dollars closer to a new pair of shoes. Get into costume by putting on your smallest, tightest cocktail dress with a G-string underneath and a feather boa around your neck—keep these last two on during the entire show. He sits in a chair with his legs slightly spread and you climb aboard facing him. As you dance, slip out of your dress and work your way around until your back is to his chest. Without taking off the G-string, reach behind you and slip him in. Instead of bouncing up and down like a

> HOW HARD IS IT? ★★
> NAUGHTY THRILLS ♥♥♥

beach ball, you swivel your hips against him as though you are dancing. Your gyrations will not only make him squirm with delight—they're designed to hit all your hot spots, too.

EXTRA NAUGHTY: If you lean forward and rest your weight on your hands while you do your thing, you can get some G-spot action.

NICE & EASY: No self-respecting lap dancer starts her moves on an already naked man. This way you can help him pitch a tent in his pants by gyrating full circle before slowly disrobing him.

Wicked Witch

> HOW HARD IS IT? ★
> NAUGHTY THRILLS ♥♥

Prepare to ride his broomstick by dressing in your most devilishly sexy witch wear. Position a magic mirror between your legs while he slides in from behind. Dim the lights so it doesn't end up looking like the "money" shot from *Snow White Does the Seven Dwarfs*, then sit back and enjoy the show.

EXTRA NAUGHTY: Have him stir your cauldron by making circular pelvic movements in opposite directions instead of just moving back and forth.

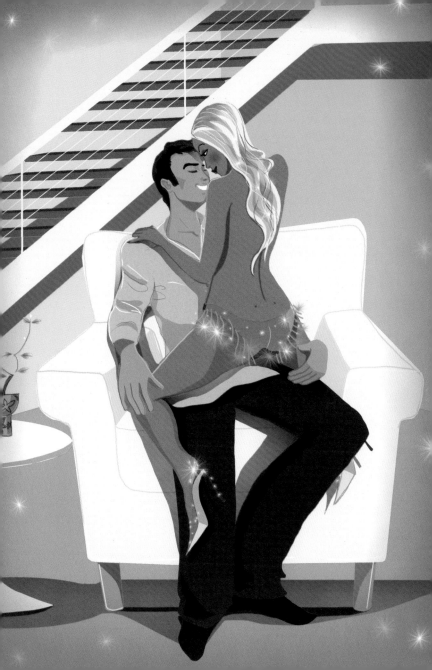

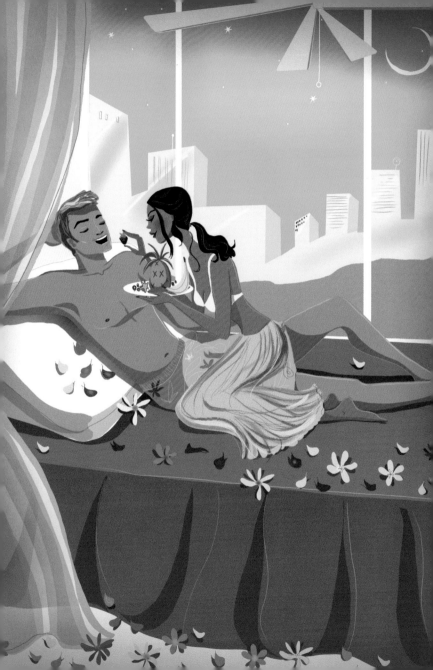

Isle Idylls

Tropical islands are just a longer way to spell S-E-X. The warm breezes, the hot sun, the scent of exotic fruits, the cute drinks with paper umbrellas... it's a sensual playground at your fingertips. As long as you have the time and money to get there—right? Actually, you can have your own tropical paradise getaway without ever leaving your house.

✳ TURN UP THE HEAT

The next hot night, get naked and stay that way. If it's not hot enough to make you want to melt into a puddle, crank up the temperature by taking a steamy shower together.

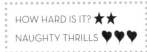

HOW HARD IS IT? ★★

NAUGHTY THRILLS ♥ ♥ ♥

✳ MAKE FLOWER POWER

In the tropics the air is heavy with the sweet, sexy scent of exotic flowers and fruit. Light lots of exotically scented candles, like mango and gardenia, to set the tropical mood. Get bouquets of flowers and scatter the petals on your bed. Your sweaty bodies will crush them as you roll around, scenting yourselves along with the air.

✳ SWEETEN IT UP

You can also add a fruit mix to your sex play—finger-feed each other bananas, pineapples, papayas and mangoes. Any drips can be licked off.

✳ MAKE IT LAST

In the tropics, there are no clocks. So forget about going straight for an orgasm and just take your time playing with each other, touching, licking and caressing. Start in the morning and finish at night.

When it is time to start swinging, jump into your bedroom hammock. If you don't have a hammock, he can substitute. He sits on the bed, resting his upper body on his arms and pulling his legs in. You settle into your man hammock by sitting on top of him, facing him, and reclining against his legs.

NICE & EASY: He slowly lowers his legs to mimic the hammock's sway.

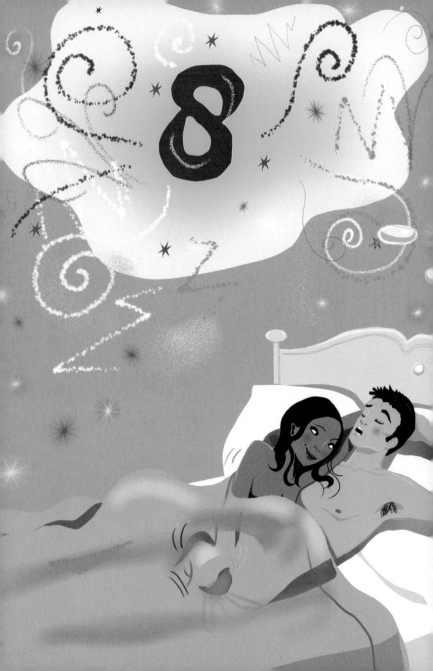

Extra Naughty

Not everyone's sexploration is going to venture to the farthest galaxies of pleasure. However, if you choose to pilot your spaceship into the unknown, always keep one thing in mind: no matter how naughty things get, as long as you are true to yourself, you'll never forfeit your gold card to the nice girl's club.

So strap yourself in for the wild ride, because this chapter is where you bring in the toys, oils, mirrors—and did someone say "straps"?

Three's Even More Fun

The Mount Everest of naughty sex—the threesome! Forming a human triangle can be a sexhilarating experience, but having a threesome is complex. He may be fantasizing about a girl-on-girl porn scene, while your image is muscular double-man action in which two guys are servicing and catering to you.

Whichever it is, threesomes are three party interactions, while sex is the contact point between two bodies. So try to make sure that someone is doing and/or receiving something to and from another person at all times. And never pay more attention to the new person than your lover. That way there'll be less chance that things will be weird afterward. Now 1, 2, 3...get on with it!

One Woman and Two Men

You sit on one man's firepole facing his feet and the other stands in front of you to get a hose down. The behind man reaches around and caresses your breasts and clitoris.

HOW HARD IS IT? *100 to make it happen,* ★★ *to actually do it*

NAUGHTY THRILLS ♥ ♥ ♥

Two Women and One Man

HOW HARD IS IT? *100 to make it happen,* ★ *to actually do it*

NAUGHTY THRILLS ♥ ♥ ♥

You and the other babe should slip into a 69 position with one of you laying on your back and the other one on all fours on top. He then kneels behind the woman on top and slides inside her.

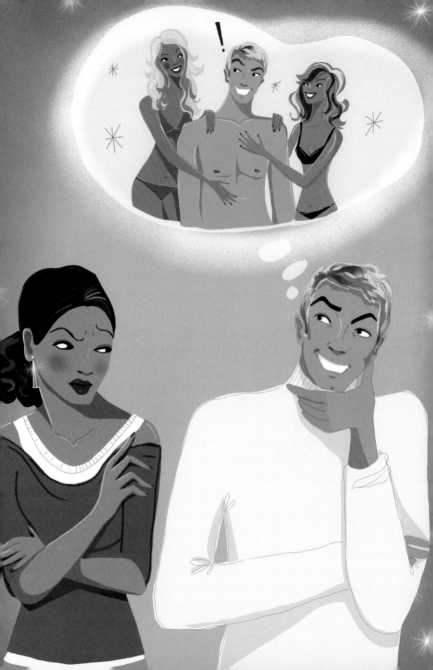

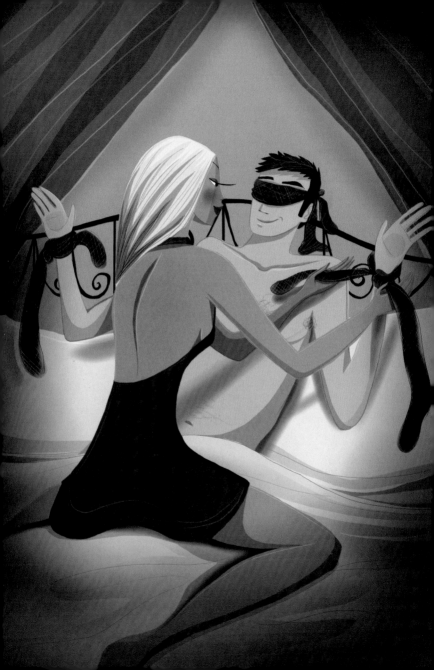

Bonds of Love

Have your lover lie back so you can tie him down with a scarf (loosely or he'll lose circulation in the wrong place). Blindfold him with another scarf so he can't see what you're doing and will not be tempted to tell you what to do. Then climb on top and lean forward to give your love nub a rubdown. Leaning backward to play bump-the-hot-spot inside your vagina and swaying back and forth will turn you into an orgasmic-drunk fool. You can also play dominatrix by holding his arms down while you ride him like your own personal love stud.

HOW HARD IS IT? ★

NAUGHTY THRILLS 🖤 🖤 🖤

Blind Passion

HOW HARD IS IT? ★ ★

NAUGHTY THRILLS 🖤 🖤 🖤

Blindfold each other and try making love in the dark—you have to feel your way. Not knowing where you'll be touched next can heighten sexual tension, and there's something about being unable to see that makes your other senses respond more intensely. When you can't take it anymore, he can roll on top of you (the easiest position to slip into blind).

Flasher

Take turns being tied spread-eagle to the bed. Turn out the lights. Using a flashlight, let light play over each other's body, highlighting each part and telling one another in great detail exactly what you are going to do to that part. Then do it.

HOW HARD IS IT? ★

NAUGHTY THRILLS 🖤 🖤 🖤

Hanky Spanky

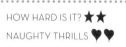
HOW HARD IS IT? ★ ★
NAUGHTY THRILLS ♥ ♥

Get on all fours on the bed while he stands behind you. The only thing that should be touching you is his penis, which is consistently going in and out. He can then lightly spank your bottom. After he spanks, he should rub it with his hand.

EXTRA NAUGHTY: He can also—lightly—grab hold of your hair from the roots and pull slightly on it. The pulling should be sensual—in other words, he shouldn't yank on your hair like he's a two-year-old trying to get mommy's attention. The mini sensation of pain will heighten your senses.

WATCH OUT!!! If you say "stop" to any of this, he should stop immediately.

Oils and Creams

Lie side by side facing each other and rub some massage cream or oil into each other's skin (there are lots of scents and flavors available from online sex shops).

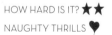
HOW HARD IS IT? ★ ★
NAUGHTY THRILLS ♥

Try to stay connected at the hips while you give each other an all-over body rubdown.

EXTRA NAUGHTY: Start by smearing some on each other's nether regions and feasting before sliding sideways.

Mirror, Mirror...

Forget overhead mirrors. Stand facing a full-length mirror with your body pressed up against your own reflection. He stands behind you and, using the mirror for support, you literally sit on his candy cane.

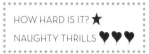

HOW HARD IS IT? ★

NAUGHTY THRILLS ♥ ♥ ♥

EXTRA NAUGHTY: Take it slow and watch yourselves melt in the mirror.

Tease Me

Too many women try to experience an orgasm as quickly as possible. Prolong your pleasure by lying on your stomach with your arms and

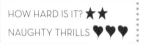

HOW HARD IS IT? ★ ★

NAUGHTY THRILLS ♥ ♥ ♥

legs spread out and, if you like, lightly tied to the bedposts. Being face-down will heighten the sensations because you won't know what's coming next. He can keep you at the brink of orgasm by building up your arousal, then climbing on top and slowly sliding in and out of you before shifting his loving attention to a less stimulating part of your body. When you do finally let go, you're guaranteed an outrageous orgasm because the release will be so exquisite.

EXTRA NAUGHTY: He should get together an arsenal of tormenting toys: feathers, vibrators and love beads, ice cubes, leather gloves (for caresses) and natural paddle hairbrushes (to lightly stroke or gently smack).

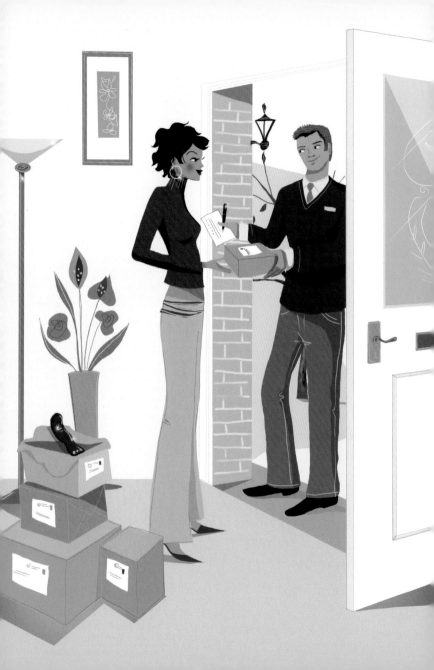

Scream Machines

There are all types of vibrators, so trying just one isn't the way to go. Think of it like buying a car: You need to test drive different models to see which one gives you the best zero-to-sixty thrill.

IF YOU LIKE IT HARD AND FAST, go for a body massager with a bulbous vibrating head that delivers powerful sensations.

IF YOU LIKE IT SOFT AND SLOW, go for a jelly rubber toy. Bonus—it's waterproof.

IF YOU LIKE IT BOTH WAYS, go for a vibrator like the Rabbit Pearl, which is designed to hit the G-spot and clitoris at the same time. Hmmm, you may not even need him along for the ride.

IF YOU WANT TO USE IT AS A COUPLE, go for a threesome-friendly strap-on like the Butterfly that will give everyone involved a bit of a buzz.

Vibrator on You

Doggy style is a great position for cranking it up with a sex toy because he and you both have easy access to your love triangle. It's easiest if you lean on your elbows and perk your bottom as high up as you can while he drapes himself over you.

HOW HARD IS IT? ★
NAUGHTY THRILLS ♥ ♥ ♥

Vibrator on Him

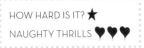

To use a vibrator on him, you should get on top, facing his feet. This way, you can buzz lightly over his balls and press against the sensitive bit of skin between his balls and bottom.

HOW HARD IS IT? ★
NAUGHTY THRILLS ♥ ♥ ♥

Backdoor

When you are ready to start your backdoor sexploration, never dive right in—start with some fingering of the area. Get in missionary, but instead of him just putting his hands on your sides, he should slide them under your bottom and give your backdoor a little finger play.

NICE & EASY: He should ensure a smooth entry by giving his finger a quick slick of saliva.

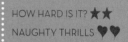

HOW HARD IS IT? ★★
NAUGHTY THRILLS ♥♥

WATCH OUT!!! Don't have him play like he's trying to hit a bull's-eye or he'll cause you more pain than pleasure (unless of course that's your thing). Go slow and easy.

When you are ready to move on to the main event, you need to be prepared. First, there's no natural juice shop located back there, so

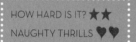

HOW HARD IS IT? ★★
NAUGHTY THRILLS ♥♥

you'll need to mix in your own. There are special lubes made specifically for the job, or just smear lots of K-Y jelly around the hole and on his penis. Second, the rectum

is not a straight tube, so anal sex is going to hurt unless you go at it at the right angle. Make sure he knows that after he has made first entry, he should aim for the belly button—but slowly, because a fraction of an inch feels like a foot when it's your bottom. You might want to wrap your fingers around the head of his penis and help to guide him slowly and carefully into the intended target.

The most popular up-the-rear position in the world is to do the hound hug, which is a basic switch-of-targets doggy style. You kneel on all fours and he comes in from

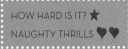

HOW HARD IS IT? ★
NAUGHTY THRILLS ♥ ♥

the back. Once you master it, you will be throwing your head back and howling with pleasure.

NICE & EASY: Lean forward and rest your upper body against a low bed or a few stacked cushions. This will take the weight off your arms and make it easier for you to relax everywhere that needs to be relaxed.

If you have done the gym work and toned your legs to steel, then you can even do it standing. All you need to do is stand to attention, bend over and touch your

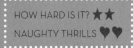

HOW HARD IS IT? ★ ★
NAUGHTY THRILLS ♥ ♥

toes. Then adjust to your lovers height with a slight squat. This simple exercise leaves as big a point of entry as you are going to get. He then stands behind and guides his cruise-liner in.

When you get really good at doing the backward boogie, try backside missionary—you lie flat on your back with your partner kneeling in front of you. To

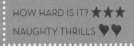

HOW HARD IS IT? ★ ★ ★
NAUGHTY THRILLS ♥ ♥

get a smooth launch onto your pad he may need to lift your pelvis a little as he goes into orbit; you can either bend your knees against your chest or rest your ankles on his shoulders—you know the missionaries never imagined this!

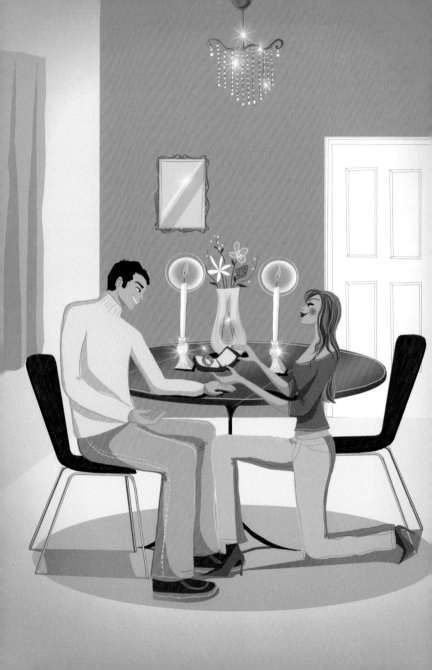

Cock Ring

What could be better then making him last longer?! On his next birthday, make sure he is one year older and better in bed. He can slip a cock ring on and then get a workout doing press-ups over your prone body.

EXTRA NAUGHTY: Because he no longer has to worry about coming to the party early, he can take his time teasing you with just the tip of his penis rubbing against your love canal before nudging against your buoy.

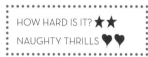

HOW HARD IS IT? ★★

NAUGHTY THRILLS ♥ ♥

WATCH OUT!!! Cock rings should not be worn for more than 20 minutes at a time—which should be enough, don't you think?

French Tickler

He slips on a French tickler and sits with his legs stretched out. You climb on top and the two of you wrap your arms and legs around each other so they are both sitting in a close clinch. Any move you or he makes will make the tickler push, bump and grind against your vaginal walls.

HOW HARD IS IT? ★★

NAUGHTY THRILLS ♥ ♥

NICE & EASY: Moving slowly so that his penis slips in and out will make sure you get the maximum sexperience from this toy.

WATCH OUT!!! Although French ticklers are worn in a similar fashion to condoms, they are not birth control devices and will not protect you from pregnancy.

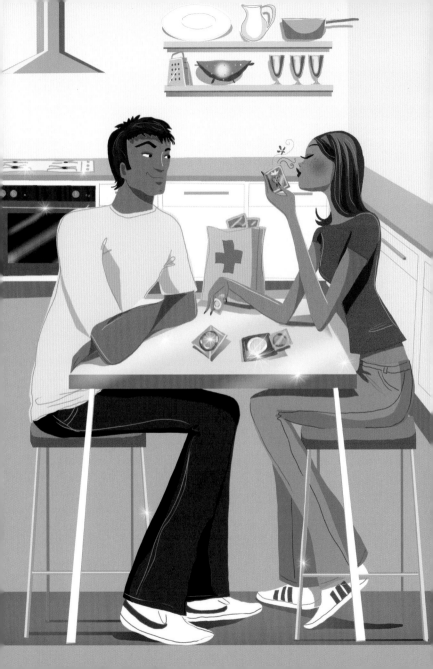

Making Safe Sex Naughty

You know how important it is to wear a condom, but do you know how to make him moan while putting it on? Here is the ultimate naughty girl party trick—slip a condom on him using your mouth.

1. Make sure to use a flavored condom that is unlubricatred and not doused with spermicide that's guaranteed to make you gag.

2. It's hard to pull this off if he isn't at least somewhat hard already. So give him the handshake to check. If he isn't, keeping shaking until he is.

3. Your mouth needs to be very, very wet. So if you have a case of cottonmouth, save this for another night.

4. Bring the condom to your mouth with the outside of the reservoir tip aiming toward you. Suck the tip into your mouth and anchor this nub against the roof of your mouth.

5. Use your hand to place the ring of the condom between your lips and front teeth.

6. Make sure that your tongue smashes any unrolled part of the condom against the roof of your mouth. This is key, because if any air gets into the condom, you could get spillage later.

7. With one hand, gently grasp his penis shaft. With the thumb and forefinger on your other hand, firmly take hold of his member just below the head.

8. Use this two finger grip to guide his head into the condom until you feel your thumb and forefinger press against your lips.

9. Slide your lips behind the ring of the condom and slowly push down so you gradually unroll the condom as you move down.

10. If you can't fully unroll the condom with your mouth, finish with your hand while you keep the mouth action going. He'll be spinning with such excitement that he won't notice you using your hand.

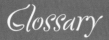
Glossary

ANAL BEADS/BALLS
Think tawdry plastic necklace. Beads that are stung together on a string and put slowly into vagina or anus so they can be pulled out during orgasm to accessorize your pleasure.

BONDAGE TOYS
Any gags, blindfolds and restraints.

COCK RING/ERECTION RING
Usually made from rubber, leather or metal, the ring goes around the base of the penis to pump up his erection for longer than usual.

DILDO
Anything that subs as a penis and doesn't shake, rattle or roll (see vibrators for this).

ESSENTIAL OILS
Oils produced by distilling certain plant materials. They are thought to have healing properties and their scents can be aphrodisiacs.

FRENCH TICKLER
Thick stud-topped condom. The nubs create a nice sensation on your vaginal entry. Ticklers, however, are primarily for pleasure purposes and shouldn't be used for STI/STD or pregnancy protection.

FRENULUM
The area on the underside of the penis, where the foreskin attaches. It's packed full of ultra-sensitive nerves.

G-SPOT
The Grafenberg spot, an elusive hot spot on the upper wall of the vagina that, when found and pressed, can make you tremble with pleasure.

LATEX BIRTH CONTROL

Latex is the material that most common condom, diaphragms and cervical caps are made of. It does not mix well with oil, which can create holes in these forms of protection within seconds.

LUBRICANTS

Emollients (oils, lotions and creams) that, when applied to the skin or to a sex toy, can increase its slipperiness, making sex a more juicy affair.

MASSAGE OILS

Scented lotions and oils that are made specifically not to be too greasy, making them ideal for sensual play.

PC MUSCLE

The muscle group that allows you to give him that extra intercourse squeeze when contracted and released. They run on the underside of your body from your pubic bone to your tailbone and can be strengthened with regular contracting and releasing. Work them out each morning while waiting in line for your morning coffee and you will have an amazing naughty squeeze in no time at all.

PERINEUM

The sensitive spot between the scrotum and anus.

PROSTATE

A potent pleasure point found inside a man's anal canal. The prostate's primary function is to aid in reproduction. It does this by secreting a fluid into semen before ejaculation occurs; this helps sperm mobility and prolongs sperm life.

RAPHE

The sensitive "seam" up the underside of the penis that helps to heat him up when stroked.

VIBRATOR

Any toy that vibrates. They come in every size, shape and texture. If you don't own one, go buy one today.

Other Books from Amorata Press

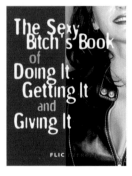

THE SEXY BITCH'S BOOK OF DOING IT, GETTING IT, AND GIVING IT

Flic Everett, $10.00

Dishing the dirty truth on everything from foreplay and oral sex to sex toys and fantasy games, this book is about being creative, spontaneous and skillful in your sex life.

THE LITTLE BIT NAUGHTY BOOK OF SEX

Dr. Jean Rogiere, $9.95

A handy pocket hardcover that is a fun, full-on guide to enjoying great sex.

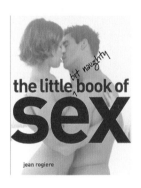

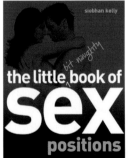

THE LITTLE BIT NAUGHTY BOOK OF SEX POSITIONS

Siobhan Kelly, $10.00

Fully illustrated with 50 tastefully explicit color photos, *The Little Bit Naughty Book of Sex Positions* provides everything readers need to start using these thrilling new positions tonight.

ORGASMS: A SENSUAL GUIDE TO FEMALE ECSTASY
Nicci Talbot, $16.95

Straight-talking and informative, *Orgasms* is a girl's best friend when it comes to understanding the physical, psychological, and spiritual factors contributing to great sex and intense orgasms.

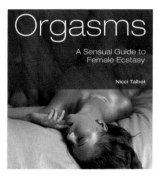

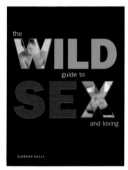

THE WILD GUIDE TO SEX AND LOVING
Siobhan Kelly, $16.95

Packed with practical, frank and sometimes downright dirty tips on how to hone your bedroom skills, this handbook tells you everything you need to know to unlock the secrets of truly tantalizing sensual play.

THE BEST SEX POSITIONS EVER!
Alex Williams, $16.95

Presents an inspirational approach to lovemaking, one designed to take readers to higher peaks of ecstasy through new and stimulating erotic moves.

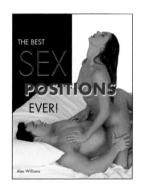

To order these books call 800-377-2542 or 510-601-8301, fax 510-601-8307, e-mail ulysses@ ulyssespress.com, or write to Amorata Press, P.O. Box 3440, Berkeley, CA 94703. All retail orders are shipped free of charge. California residents must include sales tax. Allow two to three weeks for delivery.